TOP
FITNESS
A D V I C E

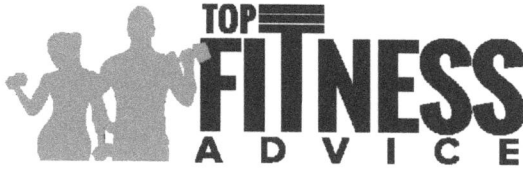

BEGINNERS GUIDE TO JUICING & SMOOTHIES

A 15-Step Guide On Juicing For Weight Loss & How It Can Help Boost Health

(BONUS: Includes Over 145 Smoothie Recipes)

LINDA WESTWOOD

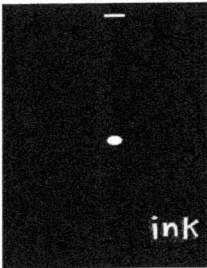

First published in 2015 by Venture Ink Publishing

Copyright © Top Fitness Advice 2019

For more information about the contents of this book or questions to the author, please contact Linda Westwood at linda@topfitnessadvice.com

Disclaimer

This book provides wellness management information in an informative and educational manner only, with information that is general in nature and that is not specific to you, the reader. The contents of this book are intended to assist you and other readers in your personal wellness efforts. Consult your physician regarding the applicability of any information provided in this book to you.

Nothing in this book should be construed as personal advice or diagnosis, and must not be used in this manner. The information provided about conditions is general in nature. This information does not cover all possible uses, actions, precautions, side-effects, or interactions of medicines, or medical procedures. The information in this book should not be considered as complete and does not cover all diseases, ailments, physical conditions, or their treatment.

You should consult with your physician before beginning any exercise, weight loss, or health care program. This book should not be used in place of a call or visit to a competent health-care professional. You should consult a health care professional before adopting any of the suggestions in this book or before drawing inferences from it.

Any decision regarding treatment and medication for your condition should be made with the advice and consultation of a qualified health care professional. If you have, or suspect you have, a health-care problem, then you should immediately contact a qualified health care professional for treatment.

No Warranties: The author and publisher don't guarantee or warrant the quality, accuracy, completeness, timeliness, appropriateness or suitability of the information in this book, or of any product or services referenced in this book.

The information in this book is provided on an "as is" basis and the author and publisher make no representations or warranties of any kind with respect to this information. This book may contain inaccuracies, typographical errors, or other errors.

Table of Contents

Would you prefer to listen to my book, rather than read it?

Download the audiobook version for free!

If you go to the special link below and sign up to Audible as a new customer, you can get the audiobook version of my book completely free.

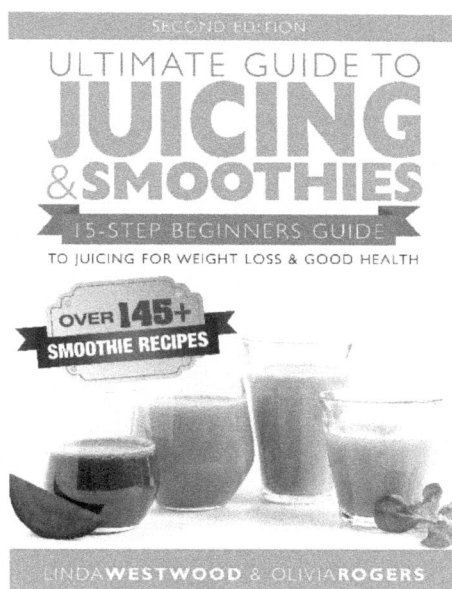

Go here to get your audiobook version for free:

TopFitnessAdvice.com/go/BeginnersJuicing

The 15-Step Action Plan to Juicing for Weight Loss & Good Health!

For your body to be healthy and functional it needs a certain amount of vitamins and minerals. Juicing is one of the best ways to give the body the nutrients it needs to function optimally. Countless cultures have collected easy to find fruits, such as pomegranates, oranges and lemons, and used them to make beverages.

The Essenes, a desert tribe in ancient Israel, pounded pomegranates and figs into a fine mash that provided subtle form and profound strength. Passion fruit was used in ancient Peru in combination with water to make a refreshing drink. So, juicing is not some latest fad of the last couple of decades.

Juicing was introduced into the modern age by Dr. Norman W. Walker, who published his book "Raw Vegetables Juices" in 1936. These days the benefits of fresh juice are well-known and the importance of juicing is on the rise because of our modern diet.

The diet most people follow is not the healthy natural diet our ancestors followed. Commercial methods of farming have robbed the soil from vital minerals and this means the vegetables and fruits lack minerals and vitamins.

Dr. Linus Pauling, who is a famous Nobel Prize winner, blamed minerals deficiencies in the diet and the soil for most of the illnesses, diseases and ailments. There is no secret that in most places the crops are raised in toxic soil and laced with commercial crop fertilizers.

Farm animals are raised in unsanitary and brutal conditions, many of the foods that are grown have been genetically altered, and livestock are feed steroids to make them produce more meat and so on. It is also well-known that the world's seafood supply has been contaminated in large parts with environmental poisons.

The average American consumes less than 20 different kinds of foods and if you combine this with packaging and storage, overcooking, shipping procedures of various countries, the processing and refinement of food, then the it is practically impossible for the average person to get enough nutrients.

Juicing is the best way to provide your body with a wide spectrum of nutrients because it condenses many different varieties of produce into one single glass.

This first section is going to go through 15 steps that will take you from being a beginner to an expert at juicing!

What You Thought You Knew About Juicing Could Be WRONG!

If you are a beginner and are maybe still a bit unsure about the effectiveness and usefulness of juicing then it is necessary to clear some of the smoke and bust some myths about juicing. There are people who claim that juicing is just a waste of money, energy and time, and that eating whole fruits is a much better option.

Of course, raw fruits and vegetables are very nutritious but due to the fiber content of whole fruits and vegetables, the nutrients also take more time and be absorbed and assimilated.

90% of the antioxidants on fruits are in the juice, not in the fiber, according to the Department of Agriculture. It is practically impossible and unpractical for people to get enough nutrients from eating raw vegetables and fruits. A person can get more nutrients from one single glass of juice than several servings of fruit and vegetables.

It is also important to keep in mind that many of the produce also goes through lots of abuse before being put into a bottle or can.

For example, when vegetables and fruits and frozen as concentrates then the chemical processes destroy a large portion of the enzymes and nutrients. So, they cannot be compared to juice made from fresh ingredients.

Discover Scientifically-Proven "Shortcuts" & "Hacks" to Lose Weight FASTER (With Very Little Effort)

For this month only, you can get Linda's best-selling & most popular book absolutely free – *Weight Loss Secrets You NEED to Know*.

Get Your FREE Copy Here:
TopFitnessAdvice.com/Bonus

Discover scientifically-proven tips to help you lose weight faster and easier than ever before. With this book, readers were able to improve their weight loss results and fitness levels. So, it's highly recommended that you get this book, especially while it's free!

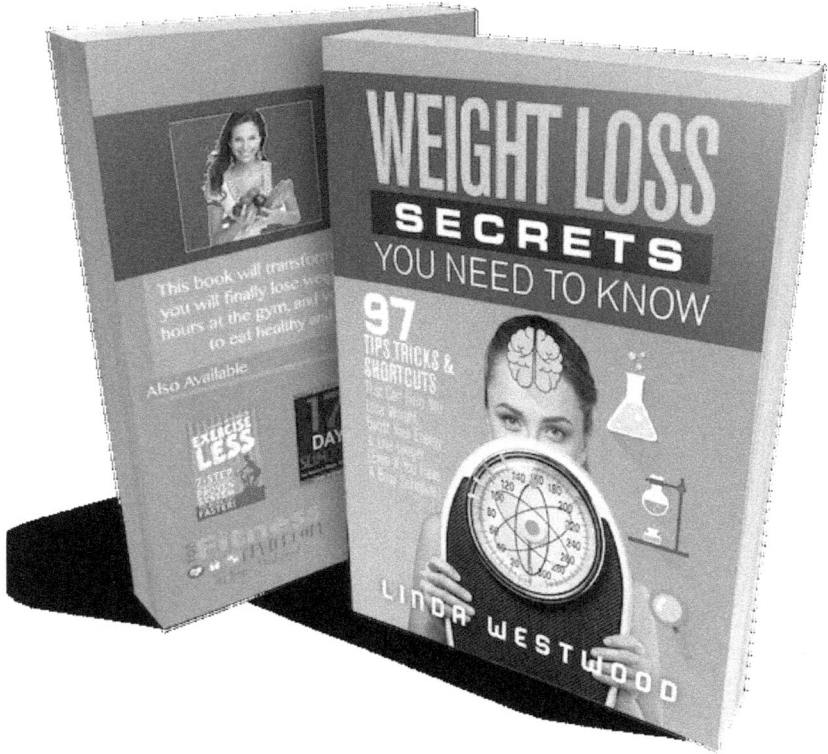

Get Your FREE Copy Here:

TopFitnessAdvice.com/Bonus

Remember the Importance of Daily Fruit & Vegetable Goals

Juicing helps people consume more vegetables and fruits. To make 6-8 ounces of fresh carrot juice, it takes half a pound of carrots.

According to an article published in September 2006 in the "Journal of the American Dietetic Association", most Americans consume well under the daily recommended level of fruits and vegetables.

One cup of fresh fruit or one cup of 100% fruit juice equals one serving of fruit. The ChooseMyPlate.gov guidelines of U.S. Department of Agriculture recommend 2 cups of fruits per day for men between the ages of 19 and 30 and 1.5 cups for women aged 31 and older; 2 cups for women 51 and older; 2.5 cups for men aged 51 and older and women between the ages of 19 and 50.

Buying A Powerful Long-Term Juicer

Juicing is very simple, fast and convenient but if you want to create high quality beverages then it certainly would pay off to learn the ins and outs of juicing and to invest a bit more money in a quality juicer.

Before you hastily buy a juicer, you first need to learn how to best take care of your juicer so it lasts as much as possible, what produce is best for juicing and what is not, what types of juicers do you actually need, what accessories you need and don't need. Doing this type of homework pays off.

Basically, a juicer is a mechanical device that can be operated either electrically or manually. It is designed to extract juice from leafy greens, fruits and vegetables. What type of juicer you ultimately buy for yourself is up to you but it is important to be aware of the different types of juicers that are on the market.

There are different types of juicers for different purposes:

- Centrifugal juicers

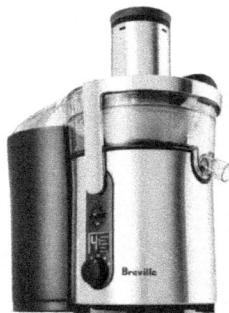

- Masticating juicers

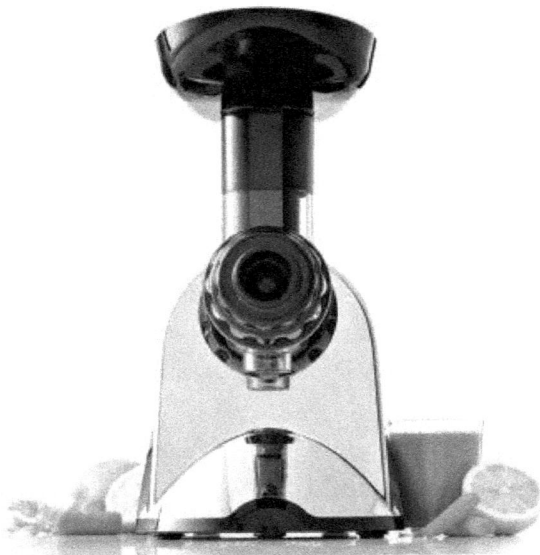

- Triturating juicers

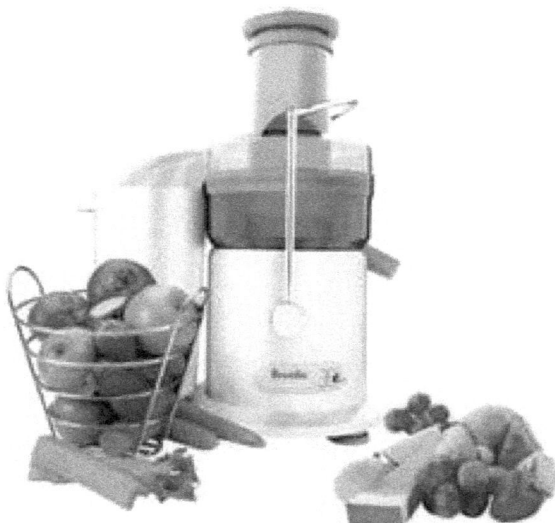

- Wheatgrass juicers

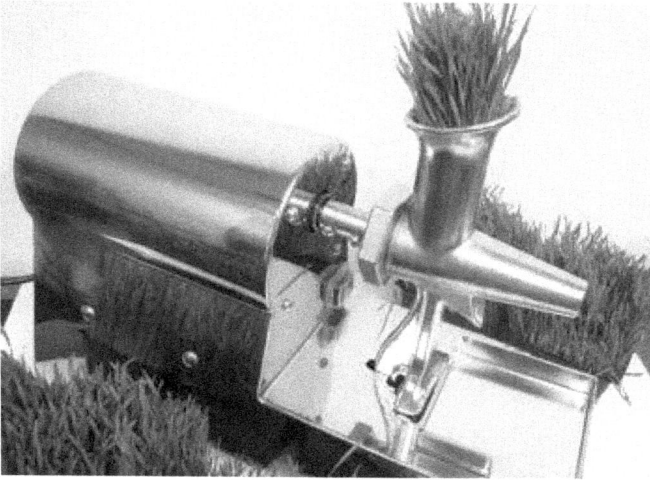

- Citrus juicers

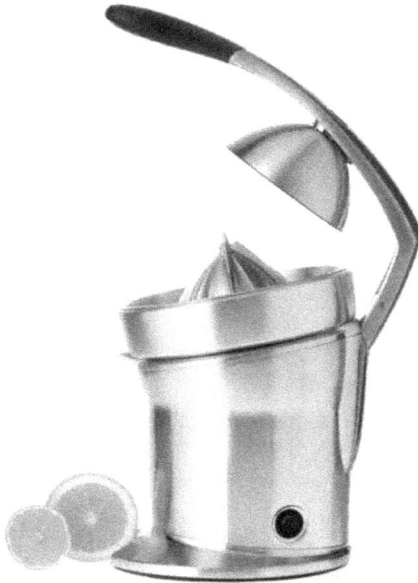

- Manual juicers

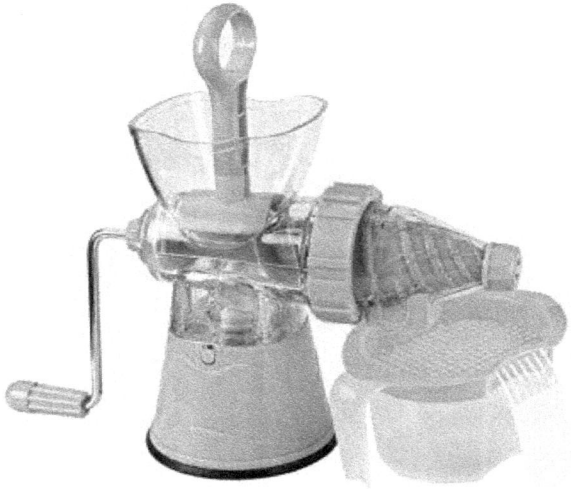

The MOST Popular Type of Juicer

Centrifugal juicers are the most popular types of juicers because they are the cheapest, oldest and have a simple design with a shredder and a strainer. The produce is shredded by a spinning basket after which the juice is forced through a fine strainer the force of the centrifuge.

The Advantage of Centrifugal Juicers

- The juice output is really fast due to the high speed and this makes the centrifugal juicer ideal for juicing on a large scale.

- There is very little preparation required because it is easy to put together and to use.

- It is inexpensive when compared to other types and models, which makes it ideal for beginners.

- This type of juicer can easily be found in department and electrical stores everywhere.

- Preparation time can also be cut short by feeding whole produce into the large and wide feeding chute.

The Disadvantages of Centrifugal Juicers

- Centrifugal juicers generally have only a 1-2-year warranty.

- The juice separates easily because it consists mainly of water.

- The juice cannot be stored for longer periods of time because the quick oxidation does not allow it.

- The yield of this type of juicers is quite low because it is not a very efficient way of juicing.

- Centrifugal juicer does not juice wheatgrass, herbs or leafy greens very well either.

- The juice itself has quite a bit of foam due to the high rate of speed that traps the air.

- Because the blades do not penetrate the produce deep enough, some of the minerals, vitamins and enzymes are not extracted from the produce.

- The motor makes lots of noise as well.

There is a bit more disadvantages than advantages but this does not mean you should not get a centrifugal juicer. It is possible to get a good quality juicer for fewer than 100 dollars and this is often the first juicer beginners buy and there is really no need to dish out lots of money for a more expensive juicer that just sits in the closet.

Once you have got the hang of juicing and have used the centrifugal juicer for some time then you can think about getting a higher quality model.

A Juicer That May ALSO Work for You

Masticating juicers work with a single gear or an auger, which is like a drill bit and with the auger comes a rotating helical screw that acts as a screw conveyor to remove the leftover pulp. The juice which is extracted from the pulp is then collected and strained through a wire mesh.

The produce inside is crushed and squeezed against the walls of the juicer once the auger starts to turn. The left-over juice is forced out and the screen, filter and wire mesh that are lined in the sides of the walls keep hold of the pulp.

Because the masticating juicers operate at a slower pace, the juice extract is not heated up and this means that much more of the vital nutrients and enzymes are left intact. A person can enjoy a more nutrient-rich juice by using the masticating type juicer.

The Benefits of Masticating Juicers

- The yield of the produce from fruits and vegetables is much higher because of the slower turning auger. The pulp of masticating juicers is much drier, which is a sign that the yield is higher. Results show that masticating type juicers produce about 15-20% more juice than do centrifugal type juicers.

- The enzymes, nutrients and trace minerals are not exposed to the heat of masticating juicers. The crushing and chewing mechanisms of this process means less foam on top of the juice and a healthier juicer for you.

- Masticating type juicers are effective and also efficient in juicing a variety of produce. They can effortlessly juice leaves, leafy greens, various fruits and vegetables as well. By using that type of juicer, you can also juice spinach, celery, wheatgrass, parsley, various herbs and other things effectively.

- These types of juicers are also versatile because the process of making juice allows a person to homogenize foods and make butter, ice-cream, sorbets, baby foods, sauces, pates and more. Some models are also able to make bread sticks and pastas for example. Due to the slower speed the masticating juicer is also more likely to last longer.

THIS Will Solve All Your Indecision Problems!

Besides the cost difference there are lots of factors to consider when buying a juicer. To be able to make the right choice, a person needs to consider all of these factors very carefully and only then make a decision.

- **Ease of use** – If you are a beginner and are looking to get your first taste of making your own juices then look for a juicer that does not require much effort and time to operate and to clean. Juicing enthusiasts are willing to spend more time on juicing but if you are just starting out then ease of use is a real plus.

- **Reliability** – If you are on the market for a juicer then check out some of the customer reviews, especially when it comes to reliability. Some juicers break down easily which requires you to change parts and that is a real hassle.

- **Multiple speeds** – It would be best to buy a juicer that has at least 2 speeds – slower speed for easier produce and higher speed for tougher produce. Cheap models only tend to have one speed. Also make sure that your juicer has electronic circuitry that maintains blade speed during juicing.

- **Horsepower** – To avoid burning out; make sure that your juicer has at least half a horsepower.

- **Feed tube** – Some juicers have a really small feeding tubes and this means you need to cut the produce into smaller pieces. To avoid this, make sure that the feeding tube of your juicer is large and also make sure the tube is easy and comfortable to use for you.

- **Output** – Obviously, you would want to get as much juice out of the pulp as possible. So, make sure that you check out the amount of juice a specific model can extract from a given quantity of produce. Ideally you would want to have a juicer that extracts at least 90% of the juice out of the pulp. Generally, the juicers that collect the pulp to an outside collector leave less pulp behind than those that collect the pulp inside the machine.

- **Versatility** – It is also important to be able to juice a large variety of produce, such as pineapple skins, carrots, beets, and watermelon rinds, delicate greens like parsley, lettuce and herbs.

- **Size** – It is also important to buy the right size of juicer for your specific needs. When you plan to make juice just for your own needs then choose a juicer with a beaker that holds a cup.

- **Simplicity** - The fewer parts juicers have the fewer parts there are to clean as well. Quite a few really good juicers have lots of parts and since the juicer needs to be washed properly after juicing then it can be a real disadvantage. It can also take some time to reassemble the juicer as well. Centrifugal juicers tend to be easier to wash than masticating juicers. Of course, you need to make sure that your juicer is dishwasher safe.

- **Continuous juicing** – It would be better to choose a machine that does not eject the pulp into center basket but rather collects into a receptacle. When a juicer has a center basket then it means you need to stop the machine and wash out the basket to be able to continue juicing.

- **<u>Quality</u>** – It is also crucial to ensure that your juicer is securely and solidly on your counter when you use it, otherwise you can find lots of juice on the floor.

- **<u>Noise</u>** – Obviously, the quieter a juicer is the better. Some brands and types are very loud and you might even need to wear earplugs when using them. More expensive models and centrifugal juicers tend to be on the quiet side.

Step 7

Making Your Juicer Go the LONG Haul

Every home appliance that is used frequently experiences wear and tear. If you want to make your juicer last for as long as possible then you need to respect its limitations, size, quirks, keep it in good working order and keep it clean as well. It is always better to be safe than sorry when dealing with machinery that has sharp blades and motors.

Here are a few tips and trade secrets to ensure smooth juicing:

- Carefully wash all of the produce before juicing. Remove mold, bruises, dings and blemishes.

- Go organic whenever possible. Organic produce is certainly more expensive but it also means you don't have to peel everything before placing the produce into the juicer and lose out of the nutrients. Non-organic produce is sprayed with pesticides that penetrate the skins, which is the largest source of nutrients in the produce.

- Always make sure you peel tangerines, oranges, bananas, pineapples, kiwifruits and grapefruits, even if they are organic.

- The leaves and stems of many produce, such as small grape stems, strawberry caps, beet stems and leaves, contain higher concentration of nutrients. So, it is best not to take them all out.

- Cut most of the produce into sections and strips that can easily fit into your juicer tube without having to jam or force them in. Of course, with experience you will learn what size works best.

- To catch the pulp during juicing, make sure you insert a grocery store-sized plastic bag in the pulp receptacle of your juicer. The pulp can be used for composting; cooking or you can just throw it away.

Step 8

What You NEED That You Thought You DIDN'T!

On top of a quality juicer, you might also need some basic equipment that you already might have in your house. Having sharp knives for peeling, coring and chopping is certainly needed. So, if you don't have sharp knives then it would be wise to make the investment.

It is also important to buy a stiff brush to be able to scrub vegetables such as carrots and beets. Having a high-quality peeler in hand is also a big plus because it allows removing the least amount of skin possible. This ensures that you are not peeling away the essential nutrients found under the skin.

There are also other accessories that make juicing much easier and comfortable. It is good to have a sieve for straining juices, flexible rubber spatulas, measuring cups and spoons. To avoid transferring any potentially dangerous bacteria into your juice, make sure you use plastic instead of wood.

Utensils, cutter boards and counter tops and many other types of equipment come into direct contact with fresh produce and therefore they need to be washed thoroughly with hot water and soap.

Also use a mild bleach solution to rinse and sanitize them. Peeled and cut fruits and vegetables should be placed on a separate clean plate and avoid adding them back on top of the cutting board.

If you have been using a wooden cutting board then it would be time to replace it with a heavy plastic cutting board that can easily fit into your dishwasher. Cutting boards that are made out of wood are porous and absorb bacteria and also allow it to grow. The same is with sponges that soak up the bacteria.

How Organic Juicing Can Boost Health EVER MORE!

Use organic vegetables and fruits for juicing whenever possible because organic produce is grown without the use of chemical biocides and synthetic fertilizers. For example, the conventional U.S. agricultural industry goes through over 1 billion pounds of herbicides and pesticides each year.

Only about 2% of this amount kills the insects; the remaining 98% goes into the air, soil, food supply and water – this includes nonorganic fruits and vegetables that people eat. So, if you buy and consume organic produce then you circumvent this health hazard.

When looking for organic produce in the store or market, look for labels that marked "certified" organic. When this label is attached to the food then this means the produce has been grown according to the strict standards of the National Organic Program. These standards include the inspection of processing facilities and farms, testing the soil and water for pesticides, detailed record keeping and so on.

Certain produce are especially vulnerable to pesticide contamination, which is another reason to buy organic. These produces include apricots, apples, cherries, bell peppers, grapes, celery, cucumbers, green beans, strawberries, green beans, peaches and spinach.

It is also best to avoid using produce that has been irradiated or subjected to gamma ray radiation to kill germs and pests and to prolong the shelf life of produce. Irradiation can lead to the formation of certain chemicals in the produce called radiolytic products that include benzene and formaldehydes.

It has to be pointed out that although the FDA has approved irradiation, then the average dose that is used to decontaminate certain produce has been measured at levels of 5 million times what a person would receive during a chest x-ray.

This radiation is dangerous and it also kills of minerals and vitamins. Not to mention that irradiating vegetables and fruits also releases a great deal of harmful free radicals.

Step 10

Learn What You Cannot Juice: Part 1

The fact is that not every fruit and vegetable – or even every part of every vegetable and fruit – lends itself for juicing.

For example, produce that have low water content are not very suitable for juicing. This includes bananas and avocados. Of course, you can still use them in your juice but you need to run them through the juicer by itself before adding them to the main juice.

Produce that do not give much in terms of yield are also not ideal for juicing. There are certain fruits that do not separate very well from their pulp: coconut, papaya, cantaloupe, strawberries, peach, honeydew, prunes and plums for example. When you want to juice these types of produce then juice them separately and add them later to the juicer mixture.

I hope that you are enjoying this book so far, and if you could spare 30 seconds, I would greatly appreciate you leaving a review on Amazon.com.

Learn What You Cannot Juice: Part 2

There are also lots of parts of different produce that cannot be juiced very well. This includes categories of stems, leaves and skins of otherwise juiceable produce that should not be part of your juice. This includes:

- The peels of grapefruit, oranges, nectarines and tangerines contain bitter oils that can cause digestive problems for some people. Lime and lemon peels can be juiced however if they are organic.

- It is important to remove the stones, pits and hard seeds from plums, peaches, cherries, apricots and mangoes. They are just too big for most juicers to handle and can easily cause damage to your juicer. Other seeds that are softer, such as seeds from lemons, oranges, grapes, tangerines, watermelons and cantaloupes won't damage the juicer.

- Seeds from apples contain tiny amounts of cyanide, a poison that can cause problems for the elderly, children and some adults that suffer from food sensitivity.

- The peels of papayas and mangos contain irritants that can be harmful when they are consumed in large quantities.

- Rhubarb greens and carrots are bitter and contain toxic substances.

- The juicer blades can be dulled when juicing large stems from grapes.

- You should not juice the peels of any produce that is grown in a foreign country where carcinogenic pesticides are legal.

- I don't have to mention that any produce that has splotches, bruises, dings and molds should not be juiced. To get a high-quality juice make sure that all the produce is freshly washed, free of any kind of blemishes and scrubbed free of dirt.

- It is also not ideal to use dried fruits, such as raisins and figs. If you really want to use figs then make sure you soak them for 8-10 hours in water.

Step 12

AWESOME Tips After You Have Started Juicing

Juice is something that is fragile and spoils rather fast. To get the most out of the juice in terms of vitamins and minerals you need to drink it right away. The juice spoils in just 24 hours, even when the juice is refrigerated.

If you are unable to consume your homemade juice right away then store the juice in the refrigerator in an opaque, airtight and insulated container. Air, heat and light will quickly turn the juice brown and zap all of the nutrients.

If you are unable to find fresh fruit for juicing then you can also substitute dry-packing frozen fruits without added sugars from your local supermarket. Some of the fresh taste and nutrients can be lost but most of them will remain intact when the produce is dry-packed.

It is also a good idea to buy large quantities of fruits and vegetables when they are locally available and freeze them for your own personal use. Drinking juice made out of frozen fruits is certainly better than drinking no juice at all.

The best way to freeze fruits is to clean, slice, peel and section fruits into smaller pieces about the size of an inch that are spread out across the baking sheet, covered with plastic and added into the freezer until frozen. Transfer the fruit into a heavy, resealable plastic bag, write down the date and make sure you use them within 2 months.

Frozen fruit can be used for juicing but canned fruit is not ideal for sure. Canned produce tends to be soft and mushy, and the fruit in cans is full of sugars or packed in sugary syrup. You should never store or refrigerate the juice of cabbages, melons and cruciferous vegetables but rather drink the juice right away or toss the left-over juice away.

Pick Your Fruits Wisely!

All kinds of fruits, whether they are grown in the ground, grown on trees or on bushes, are full nutrients and acids that heal, strengthen and cleanse the body. Fruits, also known as body cleansers, contain both complex and simple carbohydrates and they release energy over an extended time period.

Below is a list of some of the more popular fruits that people like to use for juicing purpose:

- **Apples** – They are rich in B-vitamins, vitamin C, vitamin A, biotin, folic acid and loads of beneficial minerals that support healthy hair, skin and nails. Apples also contain pectin, which is a special fiber that absorbs toxins, helps to reduce cholesterol and stimulates digestion. Apples are very versatile and this makes them very easy to blend with other juices. Apples yield about 6-8 ounces of juice per pound.

- **Apricots** - They are high in vitamin A and beta-carotene. They are also good sources of potassium and fiber. They yield about 6 ounces of juice per pound.

- **Cherries** – Rich in vitamin B, vitamin A, vitamin C, niacin, folic acid and loads of minerals. Cherries reduce the acidity of the blood because they are potent alkalizers. Due to this, cherries are used for prostate disorders, arthritis and gout. Cherries yield about 6-8 ounces of juice per pound.

- **Grapefruit** – They are rich in potassium, phosphorus, calcium, vitamin C. The red and pink varieties of grapefruits are less acidic and sweeter than white grapes. Grapefruits help to reduce skin colds, ear disorders, fever, strengthen capillary walls, heal bruising, indigestion, scurvy, varicose veins, obesity, and morning sickness. The yield is 6-8 ounces per pound.

- **Lemons** – They are high in vitamin C and citric acid. Lemons have great antibacterial properties and they are high in antioxidants. They also relieve reduce anemia, blood disorders, constipation, ear disorders, gout, colds, sore throats, skin infections, indigestion, scurvy, skin infections, and obesity. The yield is about 4-5 ounces of juice per pound.

- **Oranges** – Rich sources of vitamin B, K, C, folic acid, amino acids, biotin and minerals. Oranges strengthen capillary walls, benefit the heart and lungs and cleanse the gastrointestinal track. They help to reduce lung disorders, skin disorders, pneumonia, rheumatism, scurvy, anemia, blood disorders, colds, fever, heart disease, high blood pressure and liver disorders. The yield is about 6-8 ounces per pound.

Berries That Will BOOST Overall Health in JUST 3 Days!

- **Cranberries** – High in vitamin B complex, vitamin C, folic acid and vitamin A. Cranberries are useful because they help to keep the bacteria from clinging to the wall of the bladder, which in turn helps to prevent bladder infections. Cranberries are also used for treating disorders of the kidney, urinary tract and lungs, and skin disorders, asthma, diarrhea, fever, fluid retention and they facilitate weight loss. The yield is 4-6 ounces per pound.

- **Blackberries and blueberries** – Both of these are full of sapronins that help to improve heart health. These berries also contain minerals, vitamins C, disease-fighting antioxidants and phytochemicals. The yield is 3 ounces of juice per pound.

- **Raspberries** – They are full of vitamin C, potassium and contain 64 calories per cup. The yield is 4-5 ounces per pound.

- **Strawberries** – They are packed with calcium, iron, vitamin C, folate, magnesium and potassium – all of which are vital for the proper functioning of the immune system and for strong connective tissues. The yield is 4-5 ounces per pound.

The BEST Vegetables to Juice for Weight Loss

- **Broccoli** – Packed with fiber and also protein. It is loaded with antioxidants, calcium, vitamin C, B6 and vitamin E. It is generally used in combination with other juices because the taste is quite strong. The yield is 6 ounces per pound.

- **Cabbage** – Cabbages come in many varieties, from white to green, red and Savoy cabbage. All of the members of the cabbage family are high in vitamin B6, vitamin C and vitamin A. The yield is 6 ounces per pound.

- **Beets** – Both the beetroots and beet greens are highly nutritious and judicable. The roots of beets are full of potassium, calcium, vitamin C and vitamin A. The yield per pound is 6-7 ounces.

- **Carrots** – The ultimate vegetables for juicing. Carrots give a sweet and mild taste to various juice combos and it also tastes great by itself. Carrots are full of vitamins B, A, E, D, C and K. They are also high in sodium, potassium, phosphorus, calcium and various trace minerals. Fresh carrot juice helps to improve hair, digestion, skin and nails. The juice also has a diuretic effect and cleanses the liver. The yield is 6-8 ounces per pound.

There are also many other fantastic vegetables that can be used for juicing: radishes, potatoes, Parsnips, ginger, garlic, fennel, celery, yams and sweet potatoes, green onions, turnips, tomatoes, string beans, bell peppers, summer squash and more.

Detox Smoothies

The following section contains several detox smoothies that are broken down into three categories – breakfast, lunch, and dinner.

They contain all ingredients required to make the smoothies, along with instructions on how you can do it at home!

These smoothies focus solely on detoxing and cleansing your body through the use of the right probiotics, vitamins, and minerals.

You will notice a difference within hours and begin to feel a lot more energized and awake, rather than sleepy, lethargic, or lazy throughout the day.

Breakfast

7 Detox & Health-Boosting Smoothies

Below are 7 POWERFULLY effective breakfast drinks that are
focused on detoxing your body and boosting your health!

Although they are smoothies, you can use the tips you learned above
for juicing, as the ingredients can simply be blended rather than
juiced.

Best of all, it will provide you with an overall approach to getting
healthy!

Beetroot Sunshine Smoothie

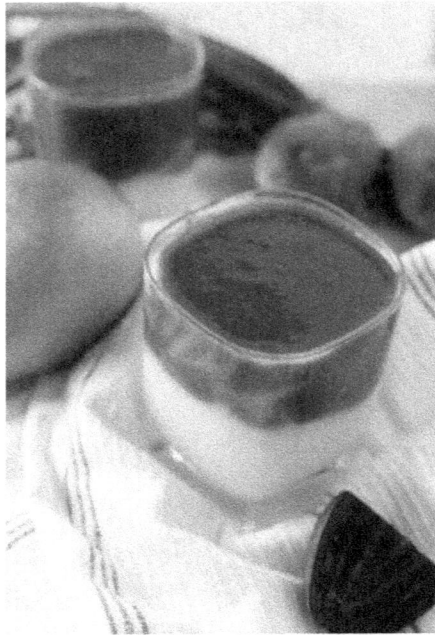

Kick-start your morning with this colorful smoothie aimed for improving your stamina. Beetroot is a great source of energy, vitamins, and minerals, so this smoothie is great for starting off your day.

Citrus fruits along with beetroot are natural detoxifiers that rid your body of toxins from the night before.

Ingredients

- 1 chopped beat (including greens)
- 3 chopped carrots
- 2 oranges peeled
- ½ cup water

Method

1. The smoothie can be made in a blender or juicer depending on preferred consistency.

2. Combine ingredients and juice/blend. Mix in liquids last if juicing.

What You Wish You Knew About Beets

- Improves sex drive
- Natural detoxifying properties
- Increase mental health

Antioxidant Smoothie

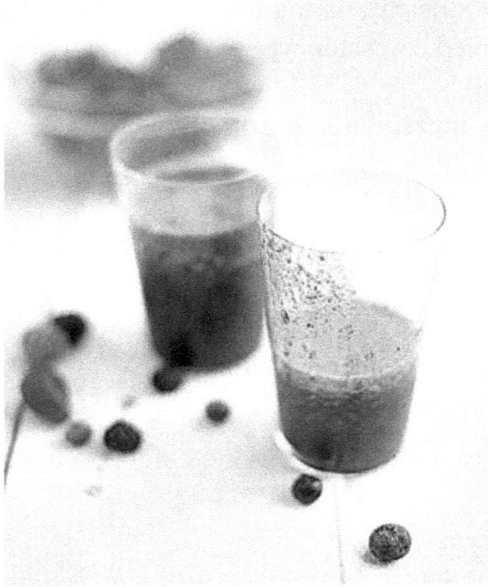

This immune boosting smoothie is great for cold winter mornings. Its main ingredient, pomegranate juice, is a nutritional super fruit. It's packed full of antioxidants and vitamins which make it great for starting the morning in winter or when you're sick!

Ingredients

- 1 cup mixed berries
- 1 banana
- 1 cup pomegranate juice
- ½ cup non-fat Greek yogurt

Method

1. Combine ingredients and blend.

Breakfast Bash

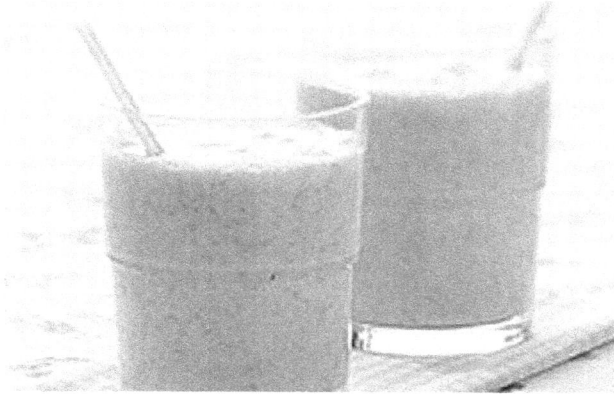

Breakfast bash is a great source of fiber with flaxseed, bananas, and raspberries. These ingredients have high levels of fiber which help fight low fiber diets that comes with drinking smoothies.

Breakfast bash is a wonderful array of fruits and veggies that help prepare yourself for the day!

Ingredients

- 2 cup spinach
- 1 cup raspberries
- 1 cup banana
- 1 cup peaches
- 1 tsp almond butter
- A dash of lemon juice
- 1 tsp flaxseed

Method

1. Combine ingredients and blend.

Lemon & Lime Detox

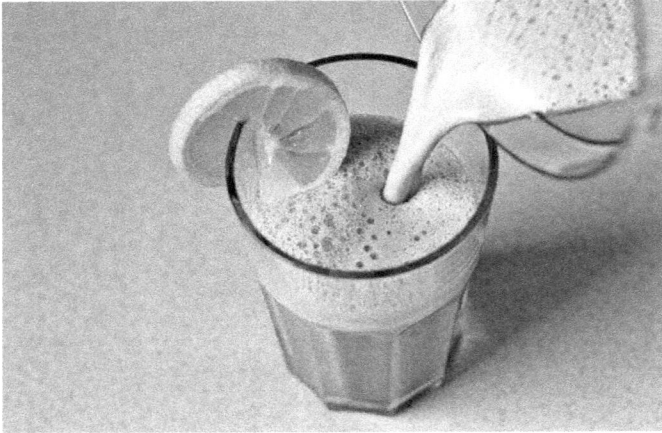

Boost your immune system with this lemon lime detox smoothie. Lemon is a natural detoxifier to help you feel great and lose weight!

Ingredients

- 1/2 medium lemon peeled
- 1/2 medium lime peeled
- 2 frozen bananas
- Juice from 1 large Orange
- 1-2 cups kale
- 1 cup water

Method

1. Combine ingredients and blend.

What You Wish You Knew About Lemons

- Lemons cause your breath to be more fresh
- Increase immune system

- Detoxifies liver
- Decrease appetite
- Balances pH levels in body
- Clears Urinary Tract

Cranberry Smoothie

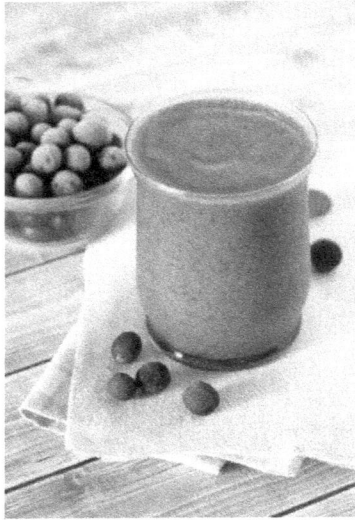

This vibrant smoothie is an exciting way to stimulate your immune system. Cranberries are high in antioxidants, which boost your immune system, so if you're feeling down and in the slumps, drink this deliciously tart smoothie and feel rejuvenated.

Ingredients

- ½ cup cranberries
- 1 celery stalk
- 1 cucumber
- 1 green apple
- 1 peach
- 1 cup spinach

Method

1. Smoothie can be made in a juicer or blender depending on preferred consistency. Combine ingredients and juice/blend.

Upbeat Beet

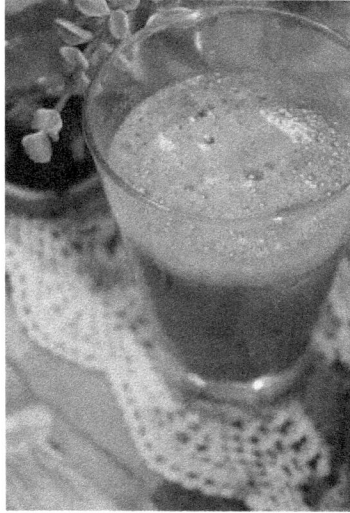

Upbeat Beet is a perfect name for this smoothie because beets are high in folate. Folate is a vitamin that has been linked to combat depression.

A lack of folate has side effects that include irritability, headaches, and fatigue. Which are all related to depression, so get upbeat with this fantastic smoothie.

Ingredients

- 1 beet
- Handful of fresh parsley
- 1 apple
- Juice from 1 lemon
- ½ inch fresh ginger
- 1 tbsp. chia seeds
- 1 cup water

Method

1. Smoothie can be made in a juicer or blender depending on preferred consistency.

2. Combine ingredients (except chia seeds if juicing) and juice/blend. Mix in chia seeds after and enjoy. If juicing mix in liquids last.

Green Apple & Pineapple Smoothie

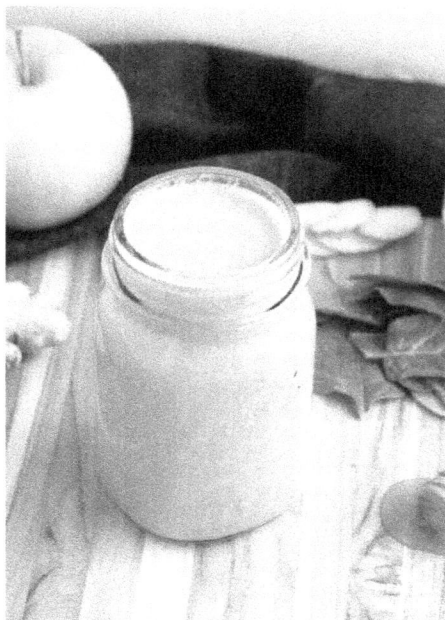

"An apple a day keeps the doctor away."

This smoothie contains apples and pineapple for flavor, but that's not all they do. Apples are known to maintain diabetes, lower cholesterol, and help with weight loss.

Pineapple is a great source of fiber and vitamins. Together, these fruits are a power couple that start off your day on a good note.

Ingredients

- 1 cup spinach
- ½ cucumber
- 1 cup kale
- 1 green apple

- 1 cup pineapple
- ½ cup almond milk
- 5 stalks celery

Method

1. Smoothie can be made in a juicer or blender depending on preferred consistency.

2. Combine ingredients and juice/blend. If juicing mix in liquids last.

6 Detox & Health-Boosting Smoothies

Below are 6 lunch drinks that are guaranteed to make you feel fuller for longer (whilst speeding up your metabolism)! They are classified as detox smoothies.

Although they are smoothies, you can use the tips you learned above for juicing, as the ingredients can simply be blended rather than juiced.

Green Grape Smoothie

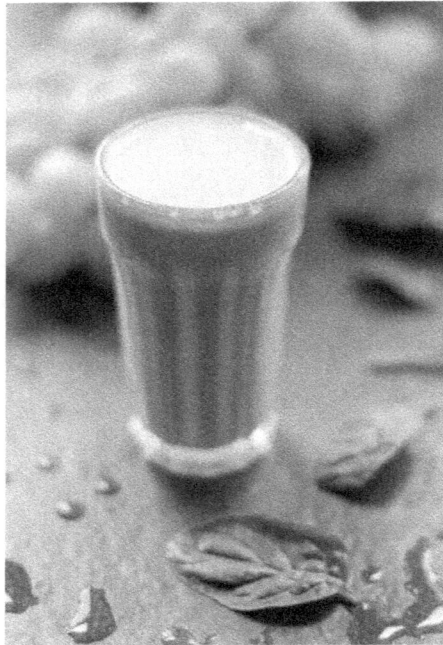

Green Grape Smoothie is an amazing smoothing great for detox as well as weight loss.

The green veggies target the detox, and the grapes target weight loss. Green veggies, like kale and spinach, are detox foods that rid your body of harmful toxins.

Grapes are found to do two things that aid in weight loss. They decrease a cell's ability to store fat and cause fat cells to disintegrate.

With the double whammy of detox and weight loss this smoothie is a great drink to add to your diet, and can have a positive impact on your health.

Ingredients

- 1 cup spinach
- 1 cup kale
- 2 cup coconut water
- 20 grapes
- 1 peeled orange

Method

1. Smoothie can be made in a juicer or blender depending on preferred consistency.

2. Combine ingredients and juice/blend. If juicing mix in liquids last.

Mixed Berries & Chia Seed Smoothie

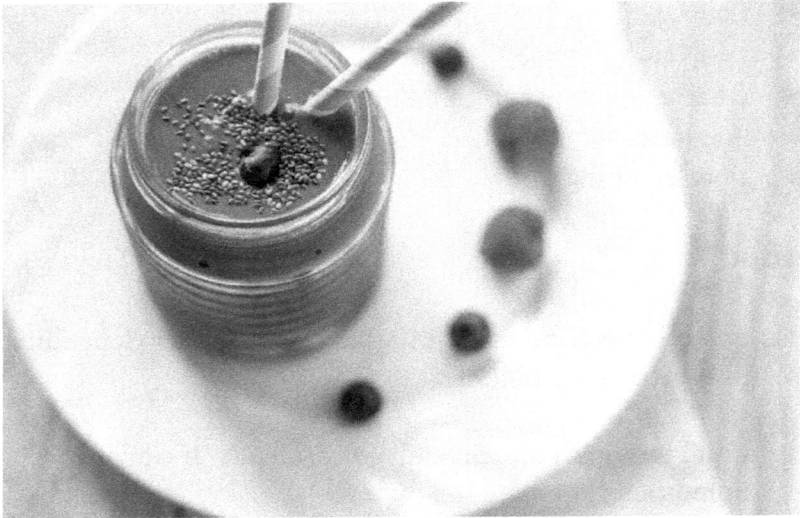

This smoothie has a massive punch with chia seeds. Chia seeds are a natural detoxifier, rich in antioxidants, and aid in breaking down carbs at a slower rate.

This makes this smoothie a great drink to add to your diet. It allows long lasting energy that keeps you fuller longer and a boost in immune.

Ingredients

- 1 cup almond milk (or milk of your choice)
- 1 cup frozen berries
- 1 banana
- 1 cup spinach leaves
- 2 teaspoons chia seeds
- ¼ cup non-fat Greek yogurt

Method

1. Combine ingredients and blend.

What You Wish You Knew About Chia Seeds

- High in fiber
- High in antioxidants
- High in protein
- The high protein and fiber content can help in weight loss
- High in Omega 3s
- Decrease the risk of heart disease and diabetes
- High in nutrients that promote bone health
- Increase exercise performance

Blueberry Blast Smoothie

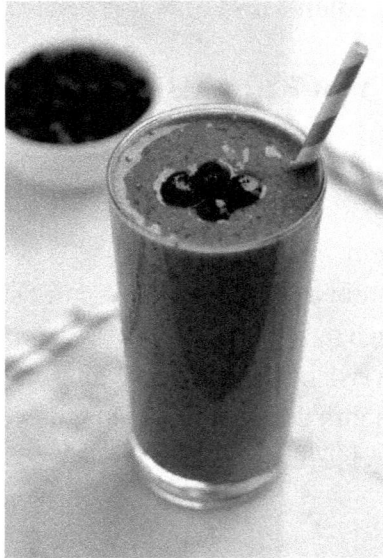

Blueberries and banana make a tasty combination in this delicious drink. Blueberries are a detox food that contains high amounts of vitamins, fiber, and antioxidants. This smoothie is a tasty lunch treat after a green morning smoothie.

Ingredients

- 1 cup blueberries
- 1 banana
- 1 cup almond milk
- 1 inch fresh ginger
- 1 cup ice

Method

1. Combine ingredients and blend.

Pomegranate Smoothie

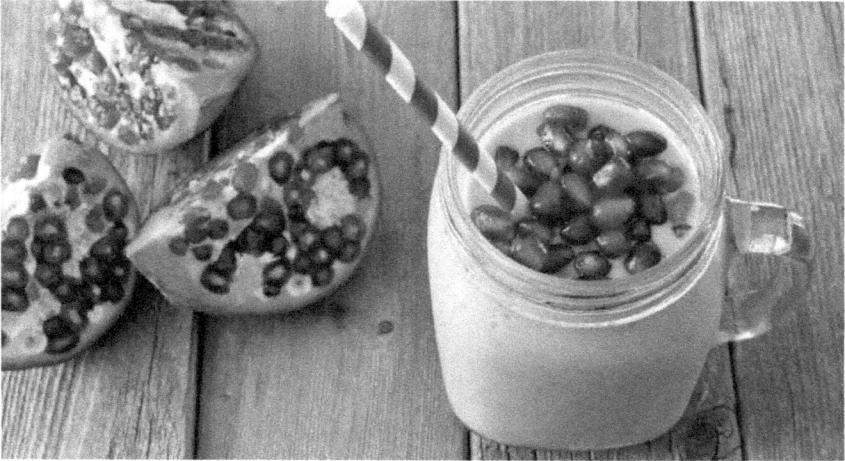

Pomegranate Smoothie is a mouth-watering tart drink packed with antioxidants.

Pomegranate juice is also great for decreasing blood pressure, and decreases risk of heart disease.

Ingredients

- 1 ½ cup berries
- 1 cup pomegranate juice (no added sugar)
- 1 cup non-fat Greek yogurt

Method

1. Combine ingredients and blend.

Green Tea Smoothie

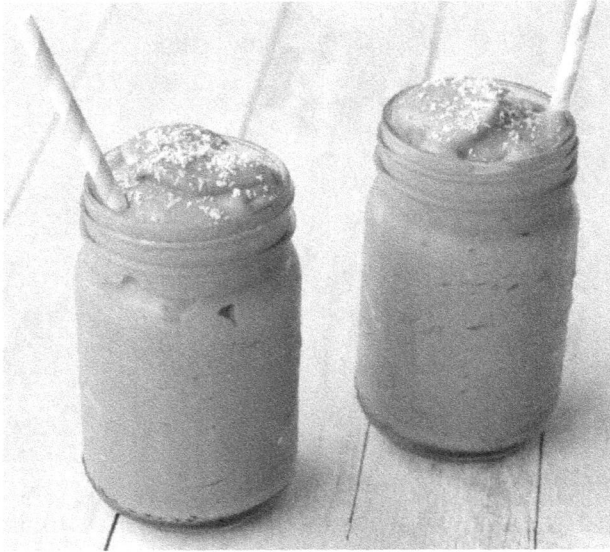

Green tea has so many positive effects for your body it's hard to know where to start.

Just to list a few, green tea is a natural detoxifier, lowers blood pressure, lowers risk of heart disease, and is rich in antioxidants. So, sit back, relax, sip on green tea smoothie, and purify your body.

Ingredients

- 2 tea bags
- ¾ cup water
- 2 cup blueberries
- 1 cup non-fat Greek yogurt
- 1 cup ice
- 2 tbsp. almonds
- 2 tbsp. flaxseed

Method

1. Brew tea bags in water and allow to cool.

2. Combine tea and other ingredients and blend.

What You Wish You Knew About Green Tea

- Increases metabolism to help burn fat
- Lowers risk of Alzheimer's
- Improves dental health
- Aids in losing weight
- Improves brain function

Sweet Green Smoothie

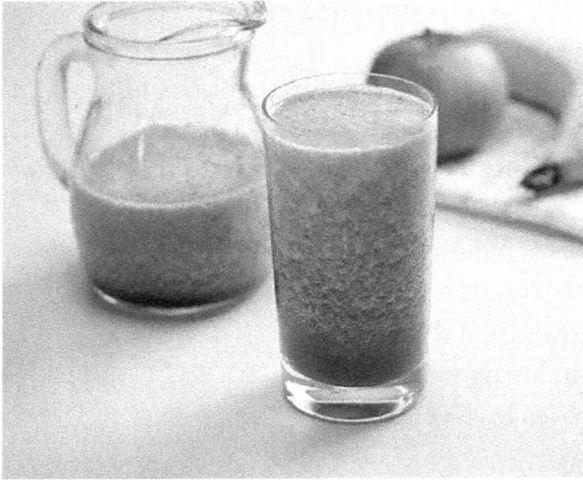

Grapes add sweetness with a kick of tart to this smoothie, which makes is delicious and nutritious. Sweet Green Smoothie is full of leafy green veggies for health, and a few fruits for taste as well as health, so this smoothie is great for people who struggle with green smoothie. Green smoothies are not always the tastiest, but by adding grapes and apples the smoothie can become tastier.

Ingredients

- 1 cup spinach
- 1 cup kale
- 2 cup almond milk
- 1 banana
- 1 apple
- 1 cup grapes

Method

1. Combine ingredients and blend.

7 POWERFUL Smoothies That Cleanse & Detox Your Body While You Sleep!

Below are 7 amazing dinner drinks that can stop night-time binges and cleanse your body while you sleep!

Although they are smoothies, you can use the tips you learned above for juicing, as the ingredients can simply be blended rather than juiced.

Best of all, it will provide you with an overall approach to getting healthy!

Sweet Potato & Orange Smoothie

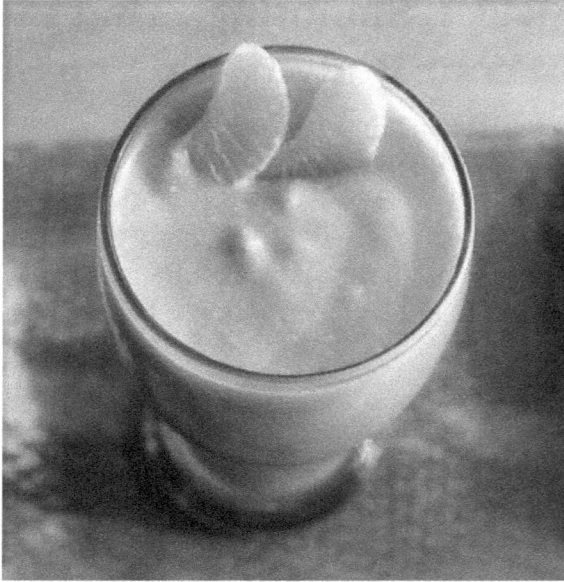

This festive smoothie is full of fiber, which is usually lacking in a smoothie diet. If you're looking for a meal replacement with fiber this should be your go to.

Sweet potato is also a superfood so its jam packed with nutrients, which will keep you fuller longer.

Ingredients

- 1 cooked and cooled sweet potato mashed
- 1 orange peeled
- 1 banana
- ¾ cup almond milk
- 1 tsp ginger and cinnamon
- 1 cup ice

Method

1. Combine ingredients and blend.

What You Wish You Knew About Sweet Potato

- Lower blood pressure
- Aid in restoring vision
- Increase immune system
- Improves digestion health
- Decrease low blood sugar episodes in diabetes patients

Green Smoothie

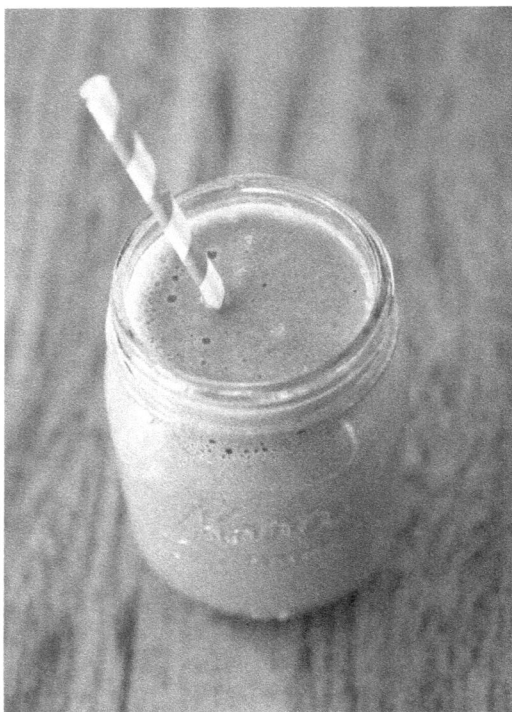

Leafy greens are a nutritional powerhouse. Full of vitamins and minerals, omega 3s, and are almost carbohydrate free.

This smoothie is great for a low carb and low sugar drink to end your day.

Ingredients

- 2 cup spinach
- ½ a cucumber
- 5 celery sticks
- 3 carrots
- 2 apples

- ¼ cup fresh squeezed orange juice
- 1 tsp lemon juice
- ½ cup pineapple

Method

1. Smoothie can be made in a juicer or blender depending on preferred consistency.

2. Combine ingredients and juice/blend (except lemon juice).

3. Mix in Lemon juice last.

Avocado Smoothie

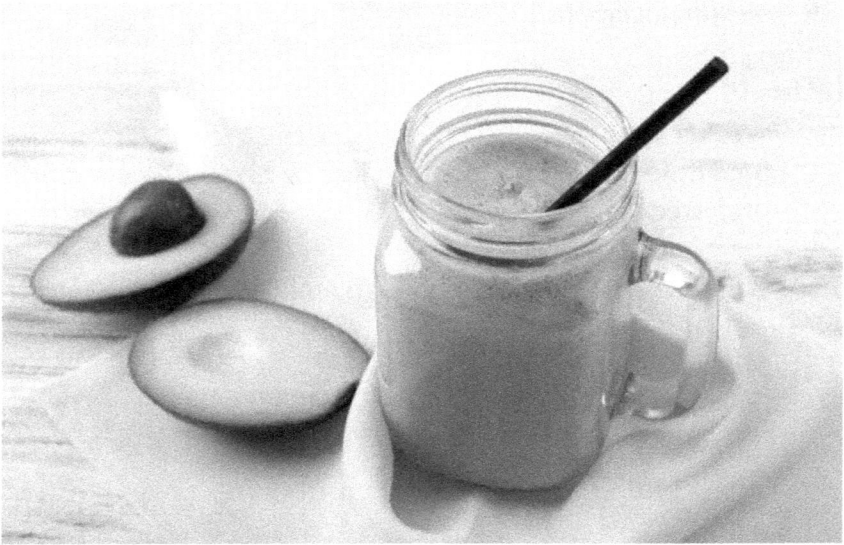

This smoothie incorporates the super food avocado, which has become a popular trend lately.

Avocado is full of antioxidants, fiber, and good fats, which are essential in a healthy diet.

Ingredients

- 1 peeled and pitted avocado
- 1 banana
- 2 cups almond milk
- 1 green apple
- 2 cups spinach
- 3 celery sticks
- 1 cup ice
- 1 tbsp. flaxseed

Method

1. Smoothie can be made in a juicer or blender depending on preferred consistency. Combine ingredients and juice/blend. Mix in liquids if juicing last.

What You Wish You Knew About Avocado

- High in potassium
- High in fiber
- Decrease cholesterol
- Aid in nutrient absorption
- Increase eye health
- Aid in weight loss

Romaine Smoothie

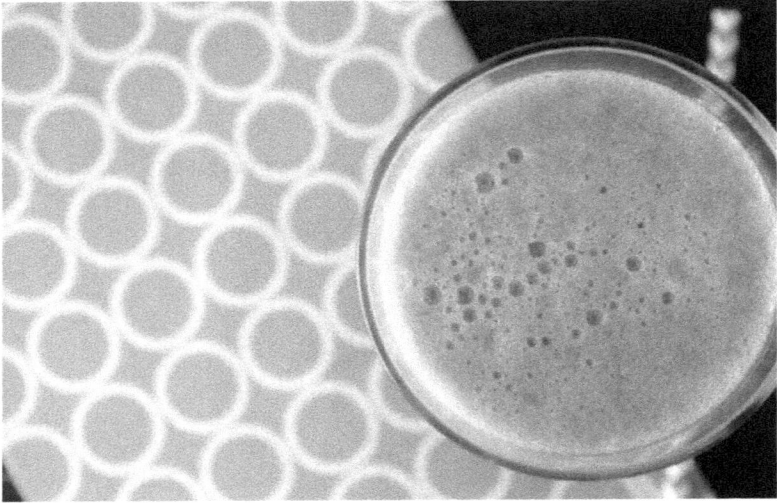

Romaine lettuce is one of the healthier options in the lettuce family. It has a darker shade of green, and therefore has a high nutritional value. This combo of avocado, romaine lettuce, and other veggies, make it a great light flavor drink.

Ingredients

- 2 cups romaine lettuce
- ¼ avocado peeled and pitted
- ½ green apple
- ½ cucumber
- Juice from half a lime
- A bit fresh cilantro
- ½ cup coconut water

Method

1. Combine ingredients and blend.

Spicy Orange Craze

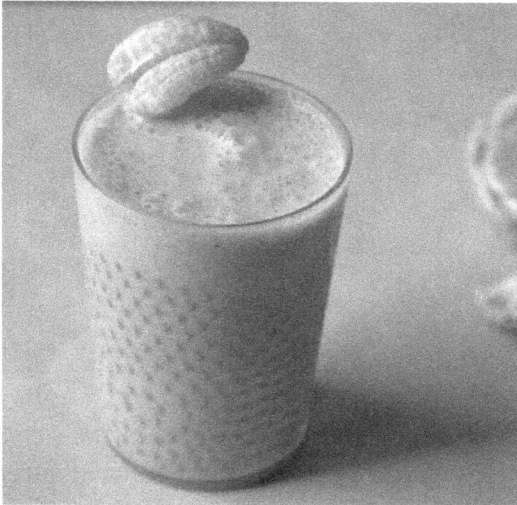

This spicy smoothie is great for revving metabolism and great for your immune system. If you're craving a colorful spicy meal this is a great substitution.

Ingredients

- 6 carrots
- 2 tomatoes
- 2 red bell peppers
- 4 garlic cloves
- 4 celery stalks
- 2 cups spinach
- 1 red jalapeno

Method

1. Smoothie can be made in a juicer or blender depending on preferred consistency. Combine ingredients and blend/juice.

Cherry Juice Smoothie

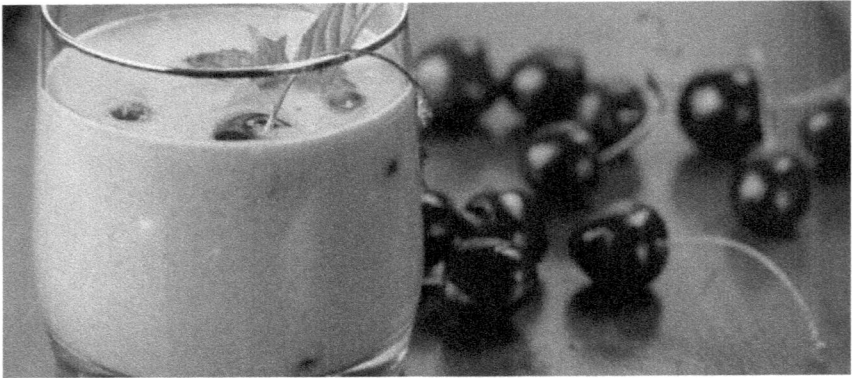

Cherry juice is another amazing detoxifier that does wonders for your body. It helps battle belly fat, fight muscle soreness, decrease risk of stroke, increase quality and length of sleep.

Sleep is also very important when losing weight and living a healthy lifestyle. So, this cherry juice smoothie is a great drink to have for dinner or an evening snack to help you fall asleep and stay asleep.

Ingredients

- 1 cup cherry juice (no added sugar)
- ½ cup almond milk
- ½ banana
- ¼ tsp vanilla
- ½ cup ice

Method

1. Combine ingredients and blend.

Cucumber Smoothie

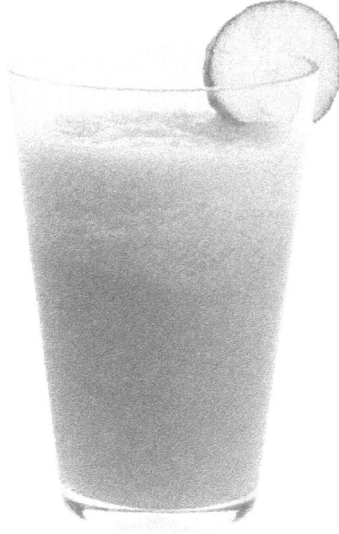

This cool and refreshing smoothie is great after a hot day. Cucumber has a unique quality to aid in regulating pH in the body, which puts this drink in our detox category.

It's great to have at night because of the minimal sugar value it has. With cucumber being composed mostly of water this smoothie is tasty and refreshing!

Ingredients

- 2 cucumbers
- 1 cup non-fat Greek yogurt
- Juice of a lime
- 1 cup ice

Method

1. Combine ingredients and blend.

Once again, thank you for reading this book, and I hope you're getting a lot of valuable information. I would greatly appreciate it if you could take 30 seconds to leave me a review for this book on Amazon.com.

Weight Loss Smoothies

The following section contains several **weight loss smoothies** that are broken down into three categories – breakfast, lunch, and dinner.

They contain all ingredients required to make the smoothies, along with instructions on how you can do it at home!

They specifically focus on boosting your metabolism and aiding in weight loss through appetite suppression (making you feel fuller for longer)!

Breakfast

7 Smoothies That Boost Weight Loss Throughout the Day

Below are 7 POWERFUL weight loss drinks that will boost your metabolism throughout the entire day and get you started feeling full and fresh all day long!

Although they are smoothies, you can use the tips you learned above for juicing, as the ingredients can simply be blended rather than juiced.

Best of all, it will provide you with an overall approach to getting healthy!

Tropical Smoothie

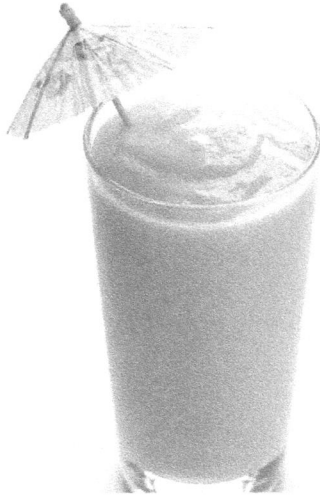

This mixture of colorful fruits has fantastic taste as well as fantastic nutrition. This smoothie has large amounts of vitamin C, other vitamins, and minerals that are great way to start your day. Kiwi also has great antioxidants in the skin, so we recommend keeping the skin on when blending this fruit to get the most out of the drink.

Ingredients

- 2 oranges
- 1 cup strawberries
- 1 tomato
- ½ cup kiwi
- ½ cup papaya

Method

1. Combine ingredients and blend.

Morning Melon & Berry Smoothie

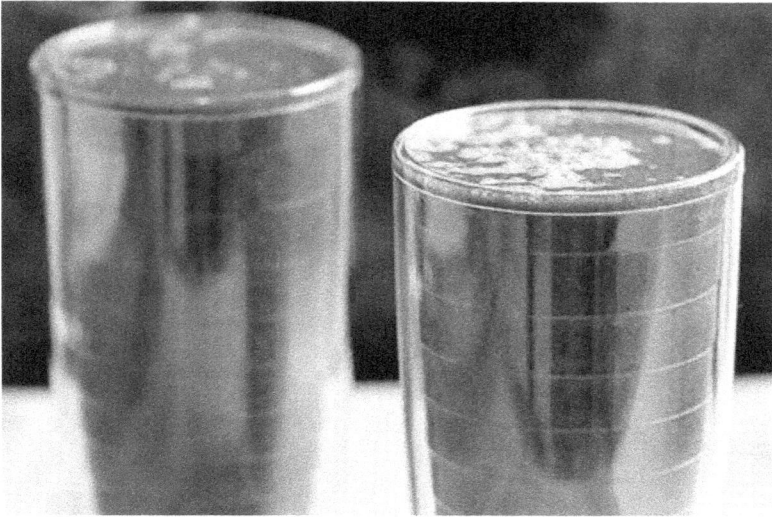

Morning Melon & Berry Smoothie is a great source of nutrients that aid in cardiovascular health as well as bone health.

This delightful combination makes for a great weight loss breakfast with the many fruits in this drink, to get the best out of this drink.

Ingredients

- 2 cups spinach
- 1 cup watermelon
- 1 cup blueberries
- 2 apples
- 1 cup pineapple
- 2 cups almond milk

Method

1. Combine ingredients and blend. Serve over ice.

Caramel Coffee Smoothie

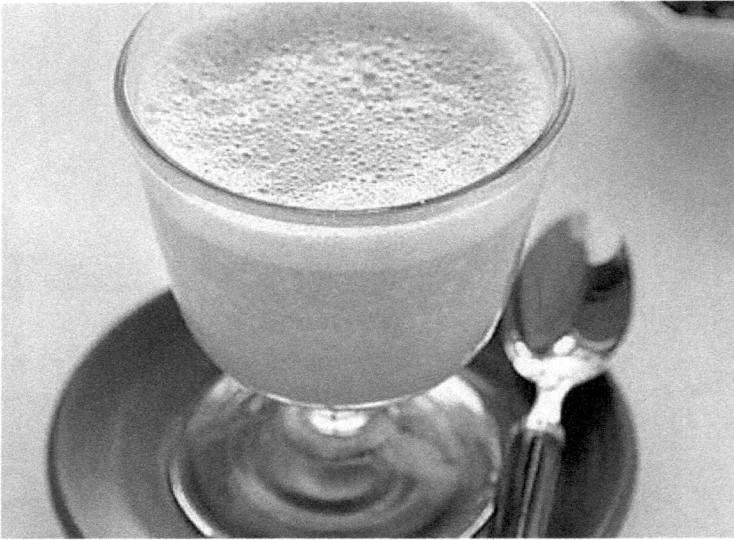

For all you coffee lovers, yes it's possible you can have coffee while losing weight. With substituting almond milk for regular milk and sugar free caramel for normal caramel, this smoothie can quench your coffee craving, but in a healthy way.

Ingredients

- 1 cup ice
- 1 cup cold coffee
- ½ cup almond milk
- 1 tsp sugar free caramel
- 1 tsp vanilla

Method

1. Brew 1 cup desired coffee and leave to cool. Combine ingredients and blend.

Mango & Avocado Smoothie

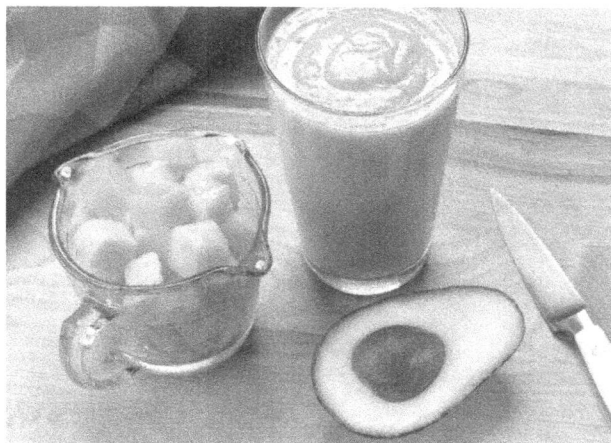

Mango & Avocado Smoothie is great for breakfast because it's high in nutritional value but sweet to get your day started. Mangos & Avocados are both super fruit full of vitamins, minerals, and dietary fiber. This smoothie will hold you over till lunch because it will keep you fuller for longer. Replace your breakfast with this smoothie on those mornings when you are feeling very hungry and want a greasy breakfast. That's why this smoothie makes its way onto the weight loss list!

Ingredients

- 1 peeled and pitted avocado
- 1 cup mango
- 1 tsp lime juice
- 1 cup vanilla non-fat Greek yogurt
- 1 cup ice

Method

1. Combine ingredients and blend.

Banana Cream Smoothie

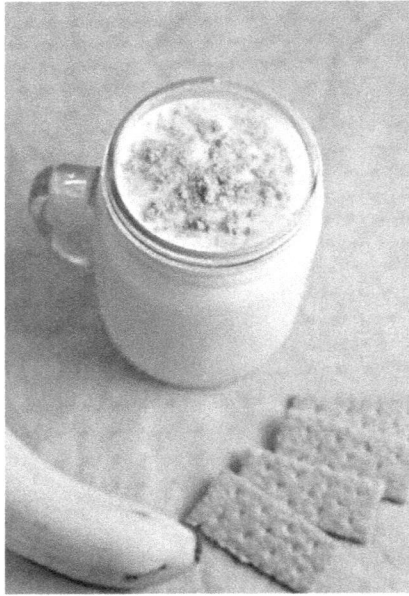

Bananas have a considerable amount of potassium and fiber to start your day with. So, for all of you with a sweet tooth, replace your sugary cereals with this smoothie.

The banana and almond milk will give you that sweetness you crave, but still giving you a healthy breakfast.

Ingredients

- 1 banana
- 1 cup almond milk
- ½ tsp vanilla
- 1 cup ice
- 2 tbsp. whole wheat gram cracker
- 1 cup non-fat Greek yogurt

Method

1. Grind gram cracker in a plastic bag. Combine all ingredients except cracker and blend. Sprinkle cracker over smoothie.

What You Wish You Knew About Bananas

- Lowers blood pressure
- Decreases chance if asthma
- Increase heart health
- Treatment of diarrhea

Fruity Smoothie

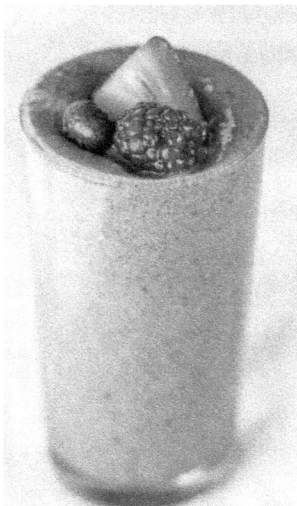

Berries are high in antioxidants; help manage diabetes, great for heart health, and great for weight loss. Berries are high in fiber and help you feel fuller longer, so this is a great breakfast replacement smoothie.

Ingredients

- 2 cups kale
- 1 cup strawberries
- 1 cup blueberries
- 1 cup raspberries
- ¼ cup almond milk
- 1 cup non-fat Greek yogurt

Method

1. Smoothie can be made in a blender or juicer depending on preferred consistency. Combine ingredients and juice/blend.

Papaya Smoothie

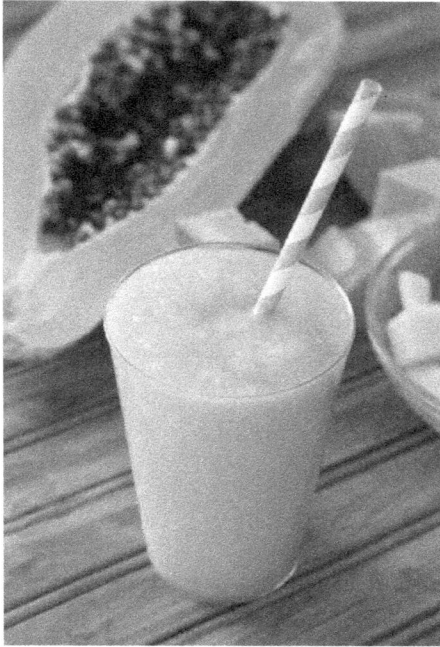

Having a smoothie that is coconut water based is great for weight loss because it's 99% fat free, cholesterol free, and contains no artificial sweeteners. Coconut water does have a bit of calories to help sustain your hunger until lunch.

Ingredients

- 1 cup of papaya
- 1 cup coconut water
- Juice from half a lime

Method

1. Combine ingredients and blend.

7 Weight Loss Smoothies That Will Stop You from Snacking!

Below are 7 effective weight loss drinks that will stop you from snacking throughout the afternoon!

Although they are smoothies, you can use the tips you learned above for juicing, as the ingredients can simply be blended rather than juiced.

Best of all, it will provide you with an overall approach to getting healthy!

Peanut Butter & Banana Smoothie

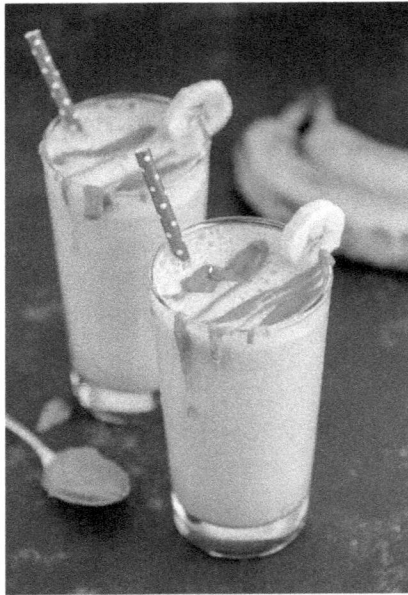

This is my favorite smoothie in this book, it's light, creamy, and delicious. If you're craving something sweet and salty, this is the drink for you. Even though it is delicious, it's so healthy.

The peanut butter gives you protein while the banana gives you potassium. This is a great smoothie to fight hunger because it keeps you feeling full longer.

Ingredients

- ½ cup almond milk
- ½ cup non-fat Greek yogurt
- 2 tablespoons creamy natural unsalted peanut butter
- ¼ very ripe banana
- 4 ice cubes

Method

1. Combine ingredients and blend.

What You Wish You Knew About Peanuts

- Heart healthy
- High in antioxidants
- Aids in prevention of colon cancer and Alzheimer's
- Aid in maintenance and loss of weight

Apple & Flaxseed Smoothies

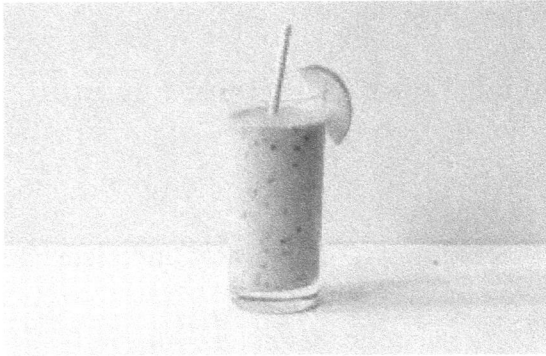

One big problem with smoothie and drink is a lot of the fiber is lost, so adding ingredients like flaxseed can fight that problem. Flaxseed is rich in fiber, protein, and antioxidants. This smoothie will keep you feeling great and full.

Ingredients

- 1 large apple peeled and chopped
- 1 tablespoon flaxseed
- 4 almonds
- ¼ cup almond milk
- 1 tsp vanilla and cinnamon

Method

1. Combine ingredients and blend.

Peachy Almond Breeze

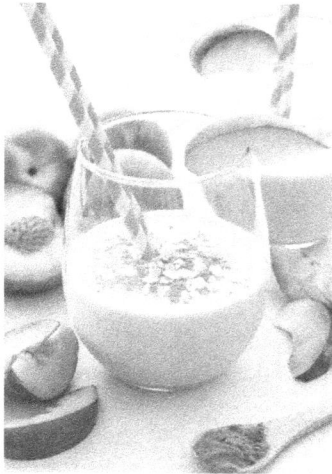

The walnuts in the smoothie are what bring a big punch. Walnuts are cholesterol free and high in protein. Combined with the bananas and spinach, this smoothie has a lot of protein. This smoothie can be used a meal replacement for dinner or lunch, but we recommend lunch because of the added fruits for taste. This smoothie will also keep you fuller longer so it can be used to fight hunger.

Ingredients

- 1 cup spinach
- 1 cup blueberries
- 1 banana
- 1 peach
- 5 walnuts
- ½ cup almond milk

Method

1. Combine ingredients and blend.

Cantaloupe Smoothie

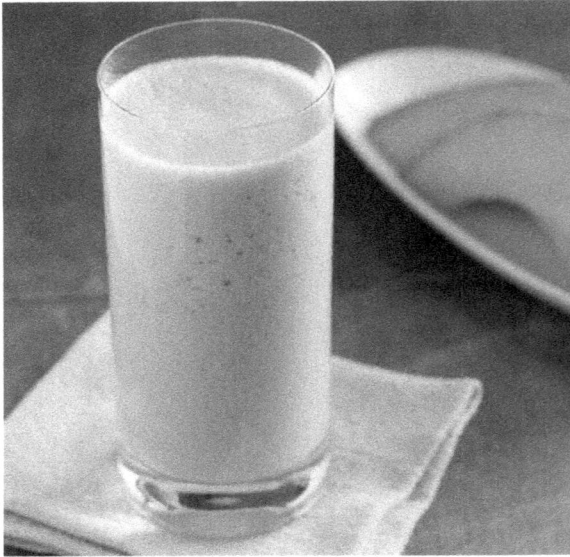

Romaine lettuce is one of the healthier options out of the lettuce family. It contains all 9 essential amino acids so it's packed full of protein and contains a massive amount of vitamin A, which aids in eye and skin health.

Ingredients

- 1 cup romaine lettuce
- 1 banana
- 1 cup cantaloupe
- 1 peach
- ½ cup coconut milk
- Handful goji berries

Method

1. Combine ingredients and blend.

Gorgeous Grape

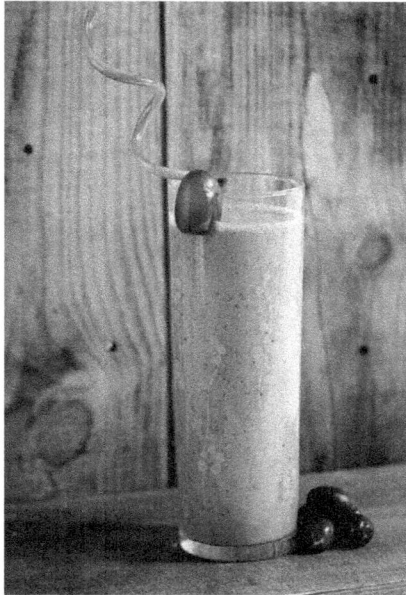

Gorgeous Grape is full of nutritional value and fiber to keep you full till dinnertime.

The kale in this smoothie gives a massive punch with its antioxidant and detox properties, nutritional value, and low calories it's a super food that gives flavor and support in your weight loss journey.

Ingredients

- 1 cup grapes
- 2 tsp flaxseed
- 1 cup coconut water
- 1 cup kale
- 1 banana
- 1 cup strawberries

Method

1. Smoothie can be made in a juicer or blender depending on preferred consistency. Combine ingredients and juice/blend. Combine liquids last if juicing.

What You Wish You Knew About Grapes

- Heart healthy
- Decrease risk of cancer
- Lower blood pressure
- Treatment of constipation
- Aid in treatment of allergy related side effects

Pina Colada Smoothie

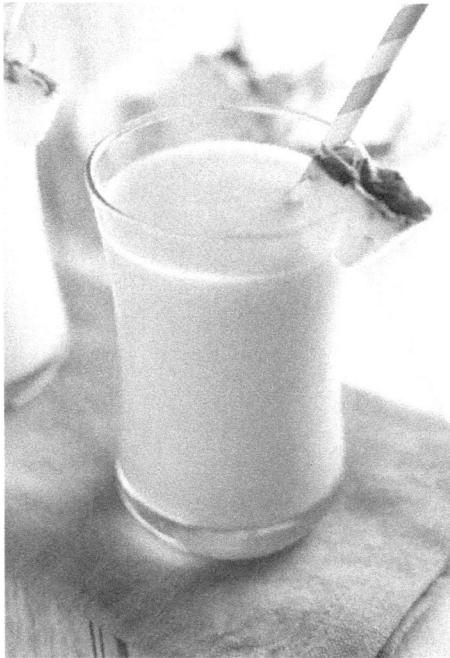

Are you girls going out for happy hour drinks, and you want to go but don't want the calories? Take along this drink to get the flavor of your favorite pina colada but without the added calories! Enjoy going out with the girls, as well as being on a diet.

Ingredients

- 1 cup fresh pineapple
- 1 banana
- 1 cup almond milk

Method

1. Combine ingredients and blend.

Cocoa & Raspberry Smoothie

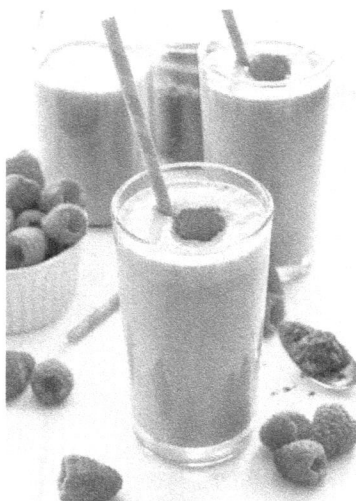

Craving a sweet treat with your lunch? Enjoy this healthy alternative to snacks and junk food. This drink gives you sweetness of almond milk and cocoa, tartness of raspberries, and creaminess of Greek yogurt. What more can you ask for? This is a fantastic low-calorie snack will have you kicking any of your greasy unhealthy snacks to the curb.

Ingredients

- 1 cup vanilla Greek yogurt
- 1 cup frozen raspberries
- 1 tsp cocoa
- 1 tsp flaxseed
- ¼ cup almond milk

Method

1. Combine ingredients and blend.

Enjoying this book?

Check out my other best sellers!

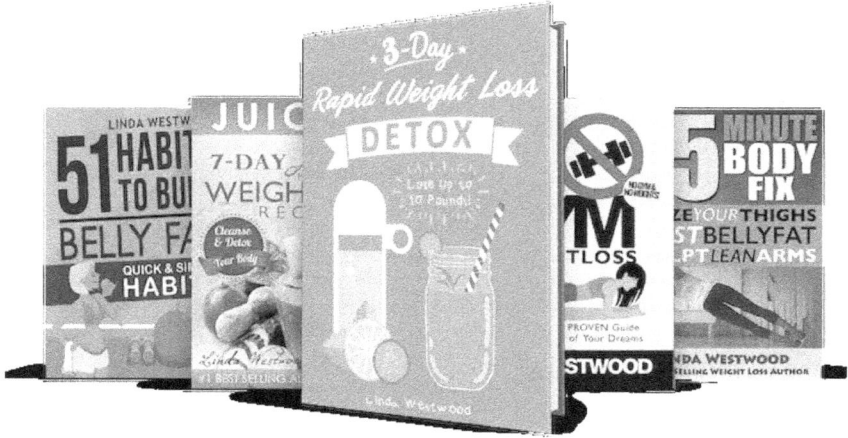

Get your next book on sale here:

TopFitnessAdvice.com/go/books

Dinner

5 Weight Loss Smoothies That STOP Late Night Binging!

Below are 5 POWERFUL weight loss drinks that are formulated to stop you from binging late at night – with a BONUS of helping you lose weight while you sleep through a few thermogenic ingredients that boost your metabolism!

Although they are smoothies, you can use the tips you learned above for juicing, as the ingredients can simply be blended rather than juiced.

Best of all, it will provide you with an overall approach to getting healthy!

Sweet & Sassy Spinach Smoothie

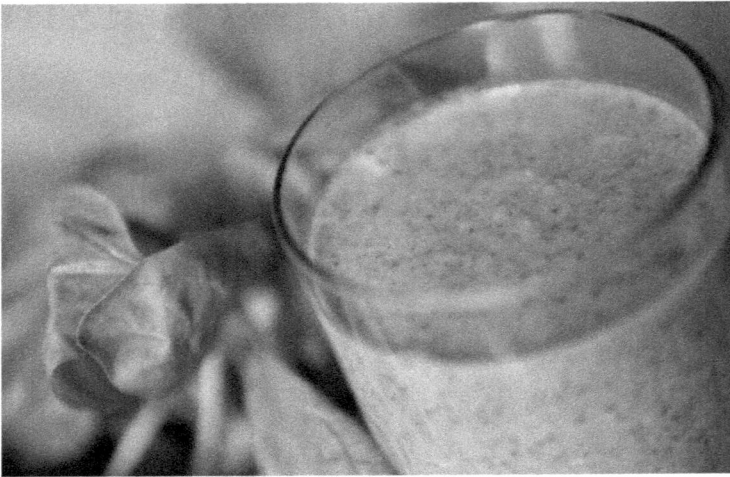

Sweet & Sassy Spinach Smoothie is a delicious way to end your evening. It's full of dietary fiber, vitamins, and minerals to hold your over till breakfast.

To maximize the benefits of this smoothie blend pears with skin on to give you that extra nutrient value.

Ingredients

- 2 cups spinach leaves
- 1 ripe pear
- 15 grapes
- ¾ cup non-fat Greek yogurt
- 2 tbsp. chopped avocado
- 1-2 tbsp. fresh lime juice

Method

1. Combine ingredients and blend. Serve over ice.

Kale & Strawberry Smoothie

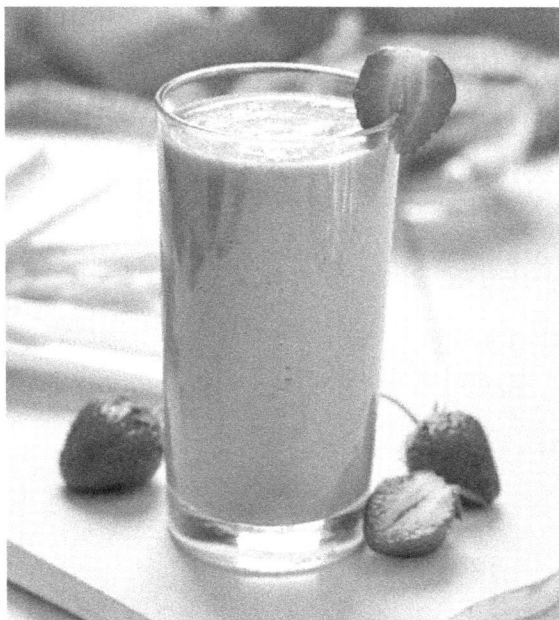

This smoothie is a light snack for you if you start to get hungry at night after your dinner.

Its sugar content is not too high, but very nutritious. With the cocoanut water and chia seeds it will give you a full feeling so you won't go snacking on unhealthy food at night.

Ingredients

- 2 cups kale
- 2 cups coconut water
- 3 cups strawberries
- 1 tsp chia seeds and almond butter
- 1 cup ice

Method

1. Smoothie can be made in a juicer or blender depending on preferred consistency. Combine ingredients and blend/juice. Mix in liquids if juicing last.

What You Wish You Knew About Kale

- Heart healthy
- Bone health
- Digestion health
- Skin, hair, and nails health

Peach Paradise

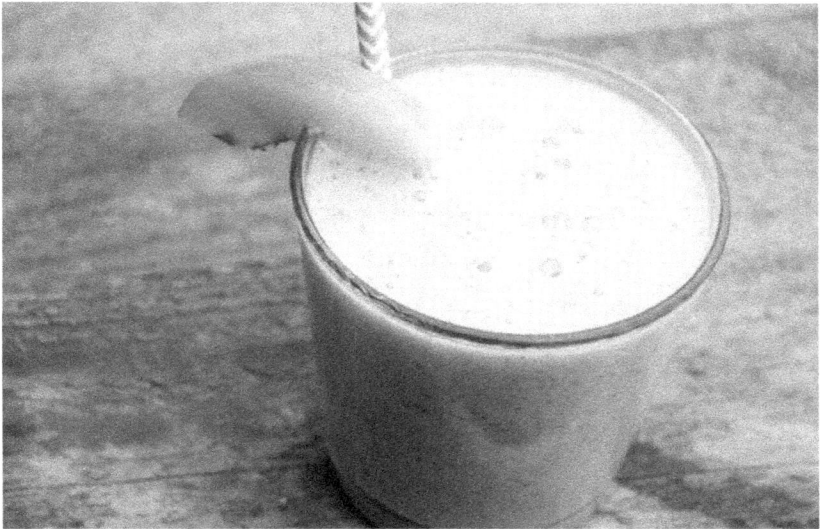

Peach Paradise is best used for an early dinner because of the sugar content of the peaches. You don't want a large sugar intake before bed so to get the best out of the smoothie use it when you are feeling very hungry for dinner but it's too early yet to eat.

A common mistake many people make while dieting is the timing of eating. So instead of spoiling your dinner with snacks, or quitting all together and going out for fast food for a fast fix to your hungry. Try this smoothie instead.

Ingredients

- 1 cup peaches
- 1 cup pears
- 1 cup green grapes
- 1 cup almond milk
- 1 cup non-fat Greek yogurt

- 2 cup kale
- 1 tbsp. almond butter

Method

1. Smoothie can be made in a juicer or blender depending on preferred consistency. Combine ingredients and blend/juice. Mix in liquids if juicing last.

Carrot Cake Craze

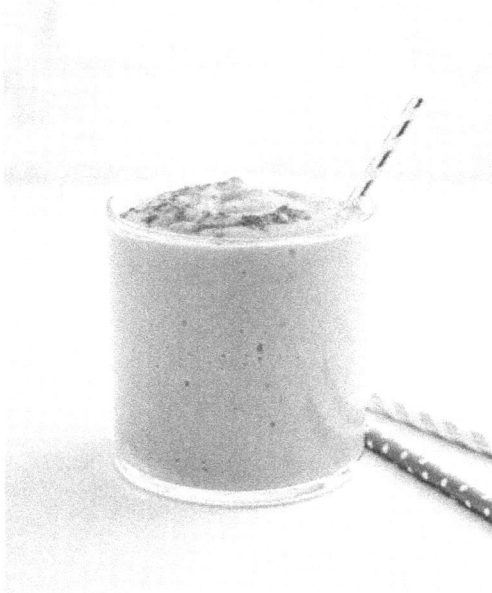

This smoothie is relatively low in calories (around 220) and in sugar, so it's great for a late dinner. Carrots are great if you're looking to stay away from a sugar drink and low calories.

You would have to eat 3 pounds of carrots before matching the sugar content in a 20-oz. bottle of cola. So, if you had a light dinner and start getting hungry again this drink should be your tasty go to.

Ingredients

- 3 carrots
- 1/2 banana
- 1 cup almond milk
- Dash cinnamon
- 1 cup ice cubes

Method

1. Smoothie can be made in a juicer or blender depending on preferred consistency. Combine ingredients and blend/juice. Mix in liquids if juicing last.

What You Wish You Knew About Carrots

- Eye health
- Skin health
- Decreases risk of cancer
- Heart healthy
- Teeth & gum health

Strawberries & Oat Smoothie

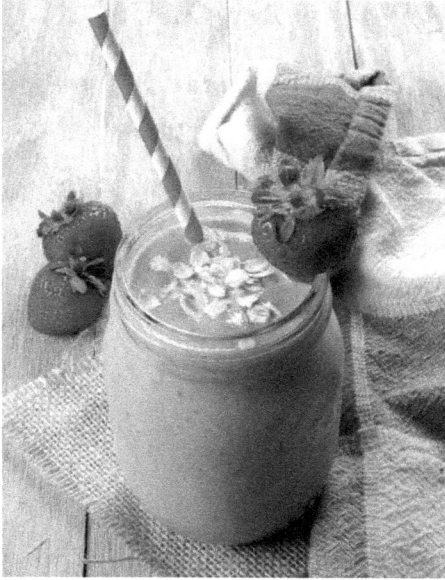

Strawberries & Oat smoothie is a great smoothie to keep you fuller longer, so you can drink this smoothie anytime of the night when you're feeling hungry.

After a long day, this smoothie is great as a substitution meal to keep you full all night.

Ingredients

- 1 cup raspberries
- 1 cup strawberry
- ½ cup oats
- 20 almonds
- 1 cup non-fat Greek yogurt
- 1 cup almond milk

Method

1. Combine ingredients and blend.

Others who are considering purchasing this book would love to know what you think. If you could spare a few seconds, they would greatly appreciate reading an honest review from you. Simply visit the page on Amazon.com.

62 Bonus Smoothies

The following section contains 62 BONUS smoothies that are all healthy and have a mixed focus on detox, weight loss, energizing, muscle recovery, etc.

They contain all ingredients required to make the smoothies, along with instructions on how you can do it at home!

Clémentine

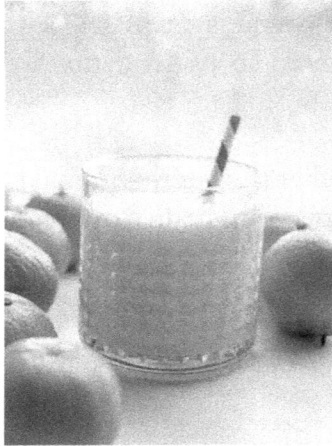

Clementines are packed full of vitamins and nutrients. One clementine gives you more than half the daily value of vitamin C in your diet. This smoothie is very tasty with coconut flakes and cocoa, but also gives you the nutrition you need. The oats and bananas give you fiber to keep you full. This smoothie is an all-round great smoothie and one of my favorites on this list.

Ingredients

- 1 cup spinach
- 1 tbsp. cocoa powder
- ½ cup coconut flakes
- 1 clementine
- 1 banana
- ½ cup oats

Method

1. Combine ingredients and blend.

Shape Up Drink

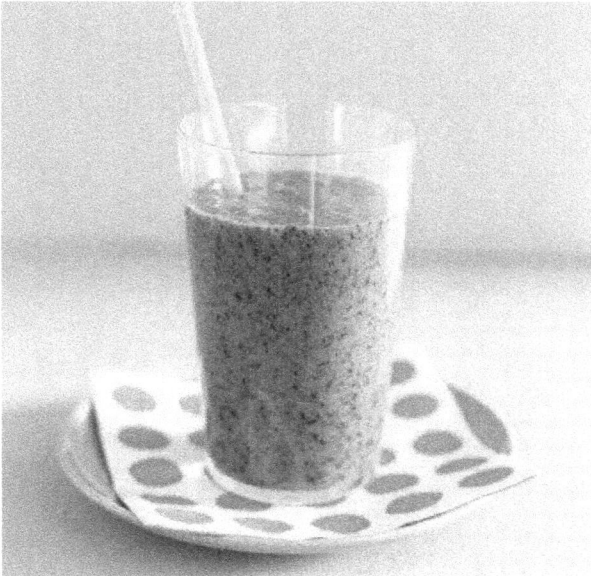

This is a fantastic drink that helps fight hunger and is great for weight loss. It stimulates your metabolism, and is great for detox as well. Feeling down and under the weather?

Try this drink to ride your body of toxins, as well as losing weight.

Ingredients

- 1 cup grapefruit juice
- 2 tsp apple cider vinegar
- 1 tsp honey
- 1 tsp lemon juice

Method

1. Combine ingredients and blend.

Metabolism Kick Mocha

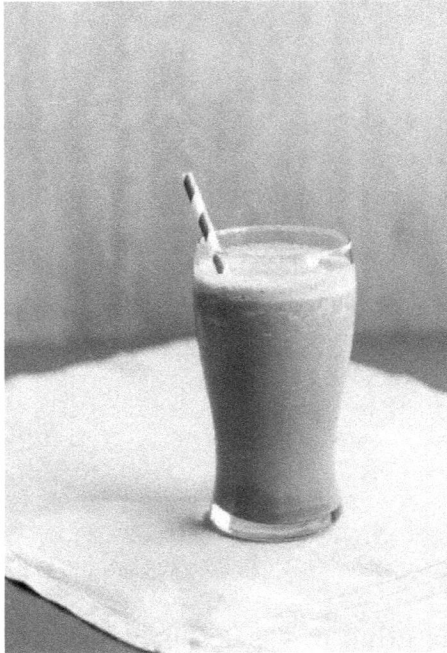

This smoothie has the chocolate taste you love but it will give your metabolism a quick kick and get it burning fat.

This is a great smoothie for breakfast or for a dessert or snack when you are craving something sweet. It has less than 300 calories and is packed with antioxidants that will keep you healthy and strong.

Ingredients

- 1 large frozen banana – To make a frozen banana cut a banana into small chunks, put it in a plastic bag and freeze it. Use the chunks in the smoothie.
- 1/2 cup cold coffee
- 1/2 cup 2% milk or skim milk

- 1 tablespoon unsweetened cocoa powder
- 1 tablespoon of nut butter like almond butter, peanut butter or cashew butter

Method

1. Blend everything together for 1-2 minutes in a blender or mix with a hand blender.

Banana Latte

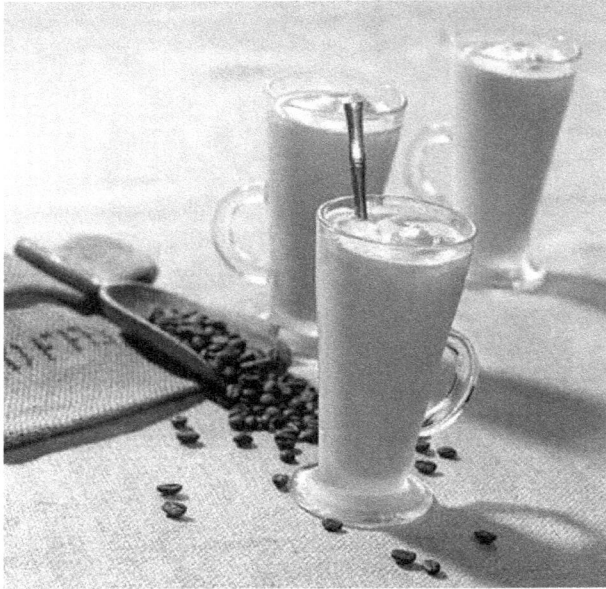

This tasty smoothie is packed with protein. Eating healthy protein will make you feel full for longer and will help you stop snacking. That will help you lose weight. This easy to make smoothie is great for anytime, especially breakfast.

Ingredients

- 1 scoop protein powder
- 1 cup skim or 2% milk
- 3/4 cup strong, black coffee
- 2 bananas cut into chunks
- 1 cup ice cubes

Method

1. Blend all the ingredients together.

Energy Booster

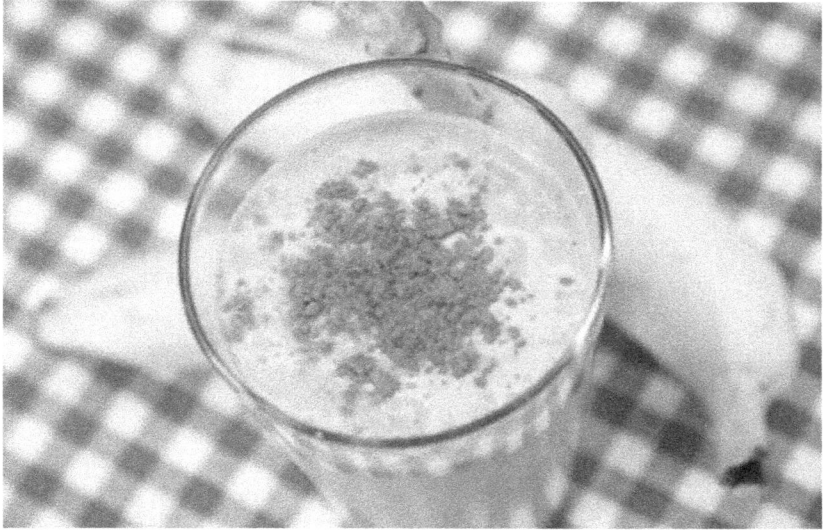

Strawberries and bananas are packed with powerful antioxidants that will wake up your body and give you the energy you need to face the day or to face a workout. This is a great smoothie to have about an hour before a tough workout.

Ingredients

- 1 cup of 2% or Fat Free Milk
- 2 bananas cut into chunks
- 1 cup of strawberries sliced or cut into chunks
- ½ cup of plain Greek yogurt
- 1 cup ice cubes

Method

1. Blend on high for one minute.

Muscle Booster

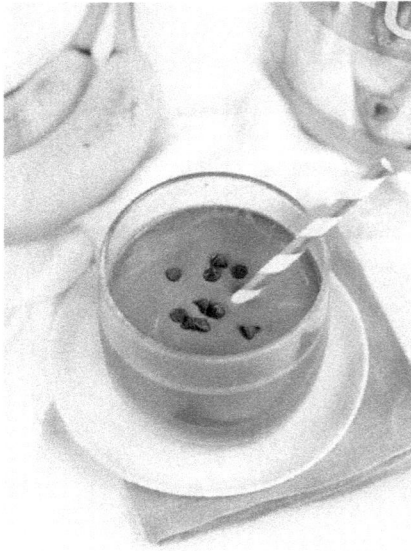

The more muscle you have the more fat you will burn. Muscle causes your body to burn fat even if you are just sitting still so building muscle will help you lose fat. If you want to increase your lean muscle mass working out and drinking this smoothie will help.

Ingredients

- 1 cup of protein powder
- 1 cup of Fat Free or 2% milk
- 2 tablespoons unsweetened chocolate powder
- 1 banana cut into small chunks
- 1 cup of cubed ice

Method

1. Blend all the ingredients together.

After Workout

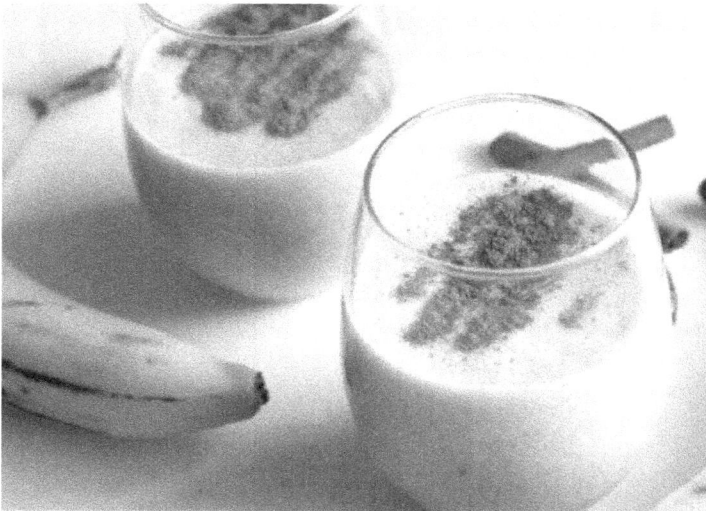

After a tough workout, you need to give your muscles the fuel they need to repair themselves and stay strong. The more muscle you have the more fat you will lose. So, after a muscle building workout like lifting weights enjoy this smoothie to give your body the nutrients it needs to heal and to increase muscle mass.

Ingredients

- 1 cup of peanut butter, almond butter or any nut butter
- ½ cup of plain Greek yogurt
- ½ cup of milk
- 1 banana cut into small chunks
- 1 tablespoon cinnamon
- 1 cup cubed ice

Method

1. Blend everything together on high.

Paleo Power

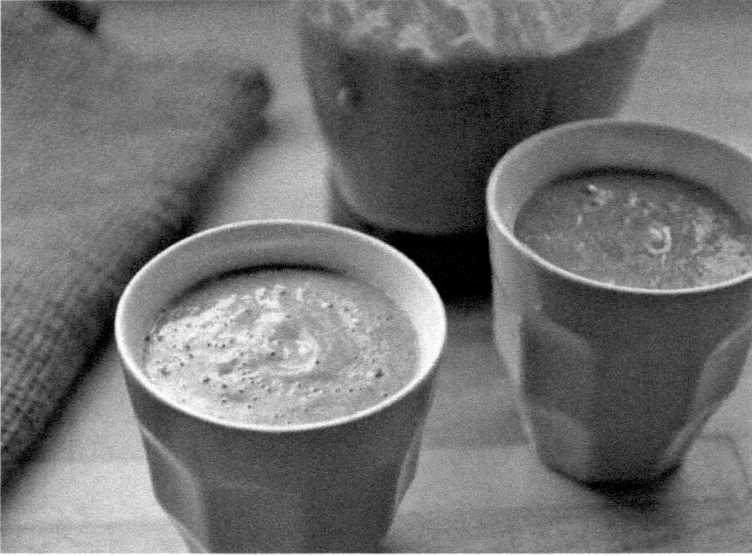

Are you trying to lose weight on the Paleo diet? This smoothie is Paleo safe and will fill you up when you are hungry but don't have time to cook a full Paleo friendly meal. Keep the ingredients for this one in a pre-measured smoothie pack so you can whip it up in a hurry on your way out the door in the morning.

Ingredients

- 1 tablespoons of ground flaxseed
- 1 cup of any frozen berry mixture
- 1 tablespoon of protein powder
- ½ cup of almond butter or any nut butter
- 1 cup of your favorite herbal iced tea

Method

1. Blend all the ingredients together and enjoy.

Energy Shot

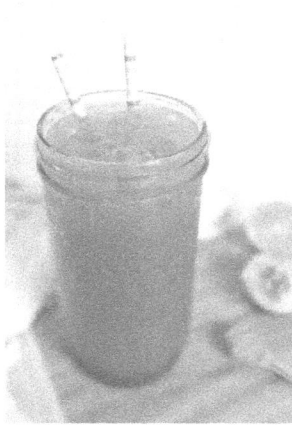

When a normal smoothie isn't going to cut it and you need extra energy to get through a busy day or a tough workout this is the smoothie that you should reach for. The vegetables and fruits along with the ginger tea will give you that extra energy shot you need to make it through the long day ahead.

Ingredients

- 1 tablespoon of lime juice
- 1 tablespoon of raw locally grown honey
- 1 pear cut into chunks
- 1 apple cut into chunks
- 1 cup of spinach diced up fine
- 1 cup of cold ginger tea
- 1 cup of cubed ice

Method

1. Blend together. Add more tea if the mixture is too thick for your taste.

Belly Buster

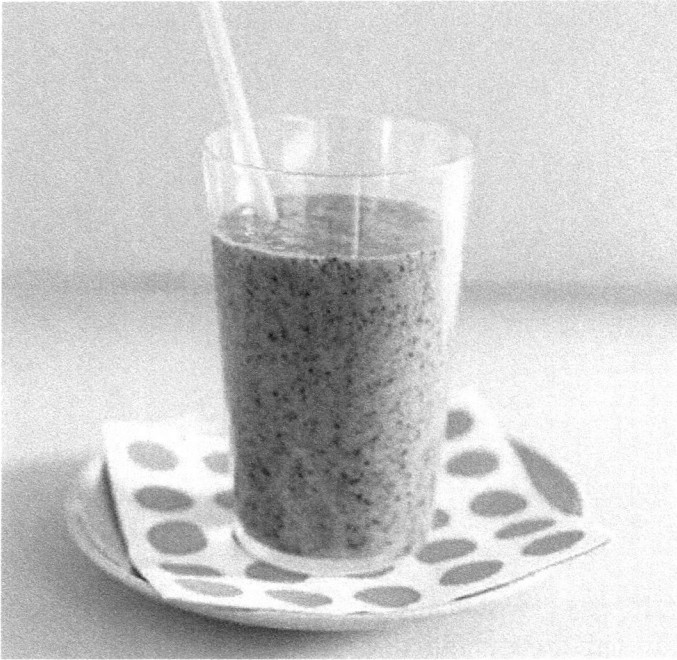

If you are trying to lose belly fat and keep from becoming bloated this smoothie will bust that bloat and help you lose fat around your waist. This is a great smoothie to have a night time snack.

Ingredients

- 2 tablespoons of flaxseed oil
- 1 cup frozen or fresh blueberries
- 1 cup of Greek yogurt
- 1 cup of low fat or skim milk

Method

1. Blend together on high.

Weight Loss Booster

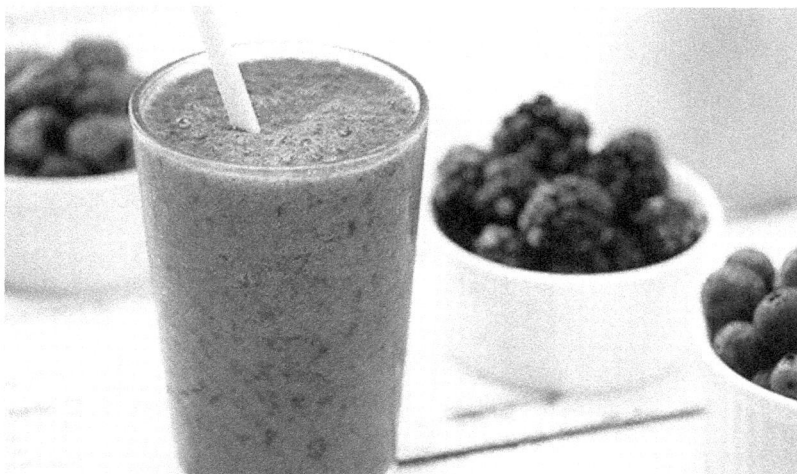

If you have been trying to lose weight but have hit a plateau and need to kick start your weight loss again this smoothie will do the trick. Replace your breakfast or lunch with this powerful antioxidant filled protein rich smoothie and you will soon be losing weight and be back on track.

Ingredients

- 2 tablespoons chia seeds
- 1 scoop protein powder
- 1 cup of mixed berries, frozen or fresh
- 1 banana cut into small pieces
- 1 cup of skim or fat free milk
- 1 cup cubed ice

Method

1. Blend everything together and use as a low-calorie meal replacement.

Breakfast Break

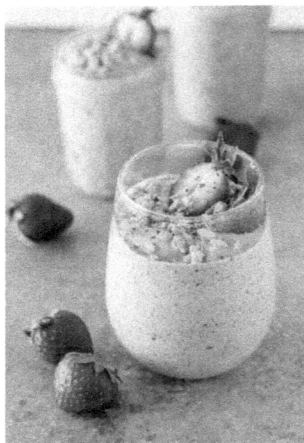

When you want to eat a good breakfast that will give you enough energy and alertness to face a big day at work or school, or a busy morning with your kids this breakfast smoothie is the one to make. Packed with protein rich nuts and healthy oats this smoothie is satisfying and delicious and will help you lose weight without being hungry.

Ingredients

- 1 cup instant oats
- 2 tablespoons of diced almonds
- 1 cup of strawberries, sliced
- 1 banana, sliced
- 1 cup of plain or vanilla yogurt
- 1 cup of milk
- 1 cup of cubed ice

Method

1. Blend all the ingredients together.

Coffee Time

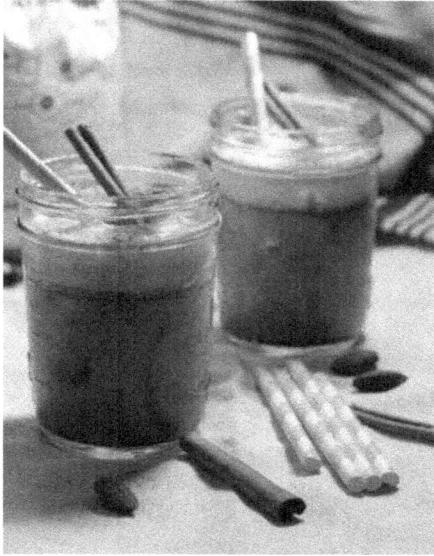

If you're craving coffee and want a quick me pick up in the afternoon this smoothie will give you energy and the feeling of fullness that you want from an afternoon snack without all the calories of chips or candy bars. Skip the vending machine and mix up this delicious coffee alternative instead.

Ingredients

- 1 tablespoon cinnamon
- 1 banana, sliced
- 1 cup of vanilla frozen yogurt
- 1 cup of cold coffee

Method

1. Blend all the ingredients together.

Sleep Tight

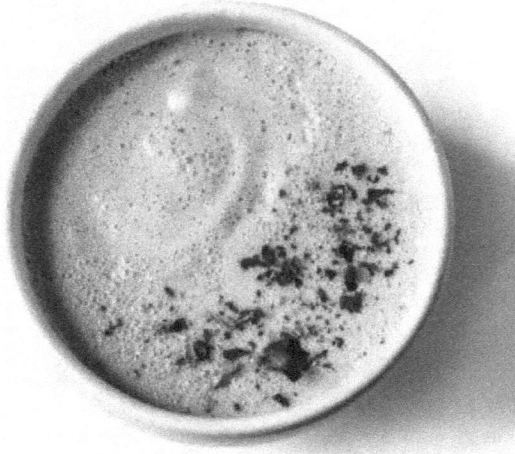

If you've been having trouble sleeping because you are hungry or stressed out try drinking this great snack smoothie about an hour before bed. It will help you relax and make sure your body keeps burning fat throughout the night without making you hungry.

Ingredients

- 2 tablespoons sesame seeds
- 1 tablespoon almond butter
- 1 cup of cherries
- 1 banana, sliced
- 1 cup of almond milk

Method

1. Take the pits out of the cherries and then blend everything together.

Stressbuster

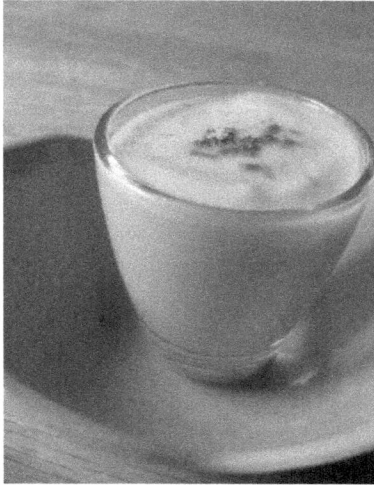

If you've been battling stress and it's making you want to eat everything in sight this smoothie can help you relax and stay on track. Don't throw away all your weight loss progress because of a tough day. Instead mix up one of these smoothies to help you calm down and keep losing weight.

Ingredients

- 1 banana, sliced
- 1 teaspoon of nutmeg
- 2 tablespoons of honey
- ½ cup of ground almonds
- 1 cup of vanilla yogurt
- 1 cup of cold Chamomile tea

Method

1. Blend together on high then enjoy and relax.

Tummy Helper

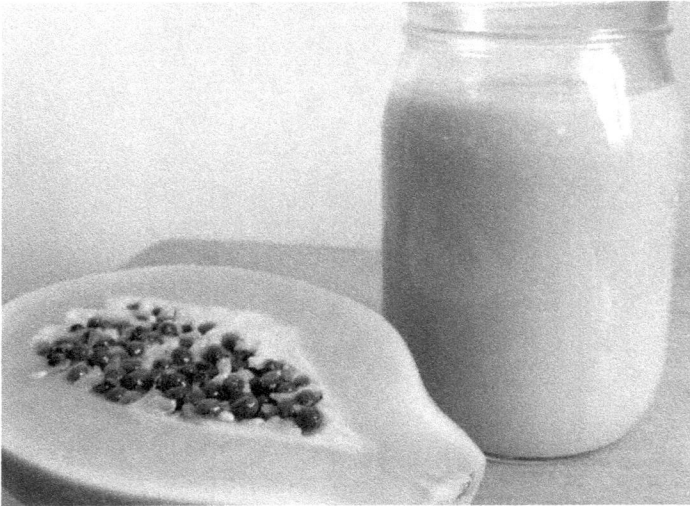

Changing the way that you eat to lose weight can result in some serious tummy troubles. If drinking smoothies has left you in distress this tasty treat will calm your tummy and get rid of any digestive troubles that you might be having.

Ingredients

- 1 tablespoon of ground flaxseed
- 1 teaspoon of ginger
- 1 pear, cut into chunks
- 1 papaya, sliced
- 1 cup of plain yogurt
- 1 cup of cubed ice

Method

1. Blend together until thoroughly mixed. Add a little honey if you want some sweetness.

Detox

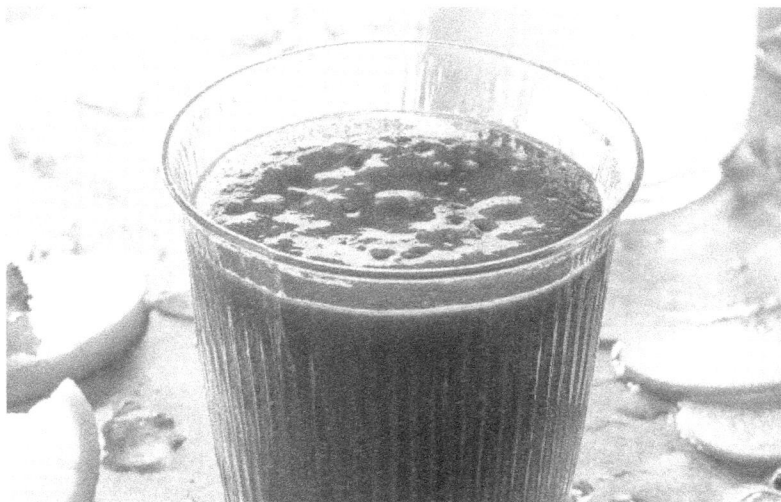

When you start a new weight loss plan, it's a good idea to detox first and get all the sugar and nasty chemicals out of your system so that you can clean your body out and then lose weight. This tried and true detox smoothie will boost your health and your weight loss.

Ingredients

- 2 tablespoons lemon juice
- 1 tablespoon ginger
- 2 apples, sliced
- 1 medium sized pear, cut into chunks
- 1 cup carrot juice
- 1 cup beet juice
- 1 cup cubed ice

Method

1. Blend all the ingredients into a healthy drink.

Skin Booster

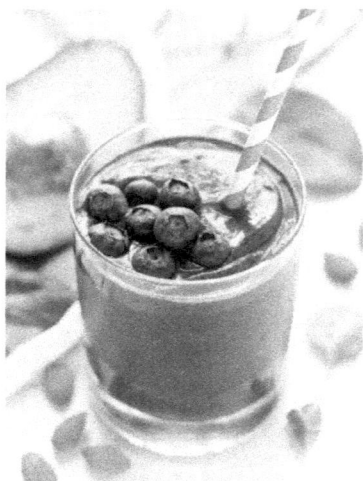

If rapid weight loss is making your skin look dull and sallow this delicious smoothie will perk it right back up again. The detoxifying foods and antioxidants in this smoothie will make your skin glow while you are losing weight.

Ingredients

- 1 tablespoon ground flaxseed
- 2 tablespoons avocado
- ½ cup blueberries
- ½ cup cherries
- 1 cup strawberries, sliced
- 1 cup vanilla Greek yogurt
- 1 cup of milk
- 1 cup cubed ice

Method

1. Blend all the ingredients together.

Immunity Booster

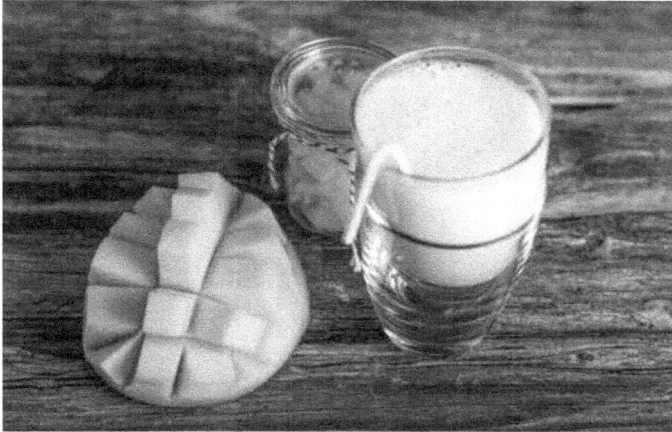

If you want to continue losing weight but you also need a little immunity booster so that your body can fight off all the germs that surround you thanks to kids and coworkers this smoothie is a great choice. You get the immune boosting power you need and a low-calorie smoothie that won't ruin your weight loss progress.

Ingredients

- 1 tablespoon ground almonds
- 1 cup cantaloupe, cubed
- 1 cup diced pineapple
- 1 banana, sliced
- 1 mango, sliced
- 1 cup of almond milk
- 1 cup cubed ice

Method

1. Blend all the ingredients together in a blender or with a hand mixer.

Spicy Cinnamon

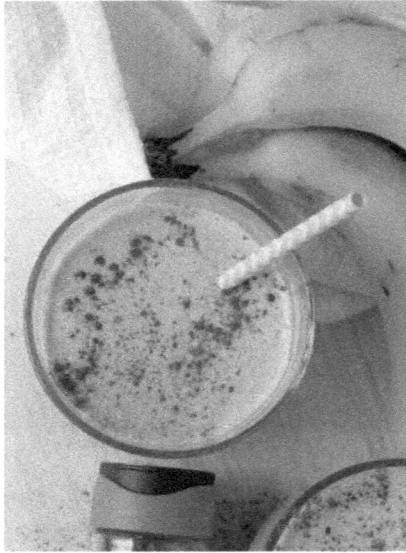

If you love cinnamon buns but are trying to lose weight this tasty smoothie delivers all the sweet spice of a fresh cinnamon bun without the massive calorie count or high fat content. This is the perfect smoothie for a weekend breakfast.

Ingredients

- 1 frozen banana, cut in pieces
- 1 cup almond milk
- 1/2 teaspoon ground cinnamon
- 1/4 teaspoon vanilla extract
- 1/2 teaspoon pure maple syrup or honey

Method

1. Combine in a blender until smooth. Add a cinnamon stick for garnish if you want.

Milkshake Style

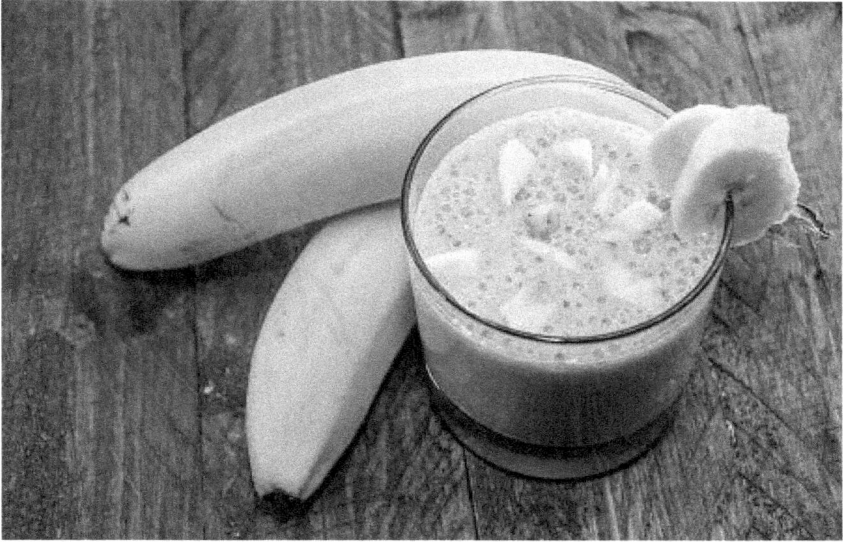

If you've craving a thick sweet milkshake but you're trying to lose weight this smoothie will give you the best of both worlds. You'll get the thick, sweet, rich taste you are craving in a smoothie that has less than half the calories of a traditional ice cream milkshake.

Ingredients

- 1 banana, cut into pieces
- 1 cup vanilla frozen yogurt
- 2 tablespoons of sweetened chocolate powder
- ½ teaspoon of vanilla extract
- 1 cup milk
- 1 cup cubed ice

Method

1. Blend together until frothy and enjoy.

Spinach Breakfast

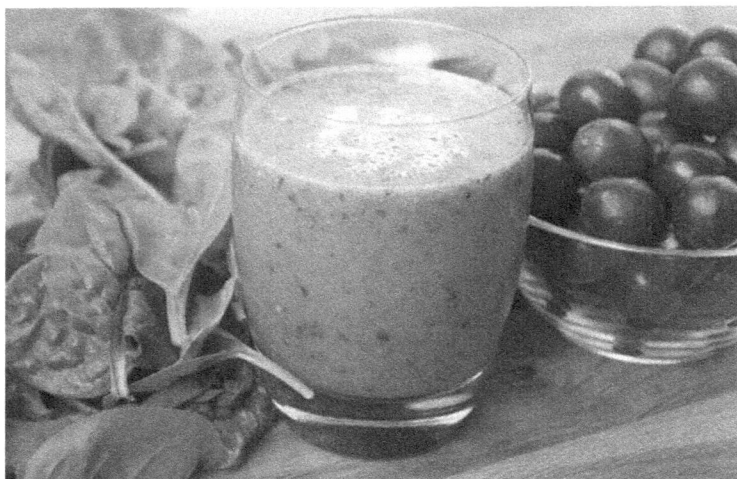

You might think that spinach doesn't sound too appealing for breakfast but spinach is the perfect breakfast food. It's packed with healthy antioxidants that will give you energy and give you a great immune system boost. It's also nutritious and filling so that you will have energy to get through your morning. Try it and see. You'll love it.

Ingredients

- 2 cups spinach leaves, chopped up small
- 1 ripe pear, peeled and cubed
- 15 green or red grapes, make sure they are seedless
- 1 cup fat-free plain Greek yogurt
- 2 tablespoons chopped avocado
- 1 or 2 tablespoons fresh lime juice

Method

1. Blend and enjoy.

Apple Flaxseed

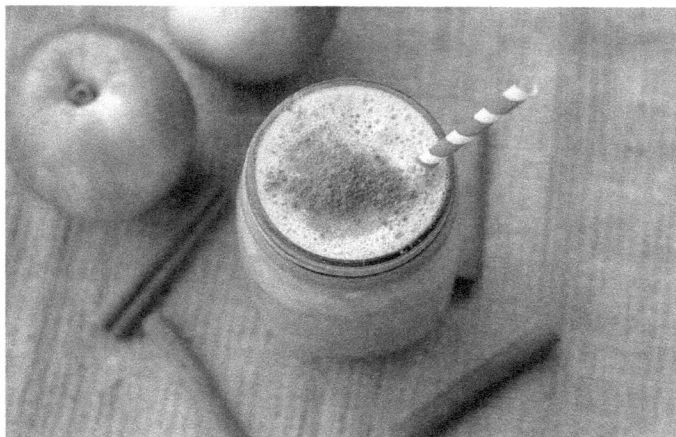

This super healthy smoothie is the perfect start to the day. The delicious taste of apples and cinnamon will get you moving and the healthy coconut water and flaxseed will keep you full until lunch. Try this tasty morning smoothie and you'll be hooked.

Ingredients

- ½ cup ounces coconut water
- 1 tablespoon of ground almonds
- 1 teaspoon vanilla extract
- 1 teaspoon cinnamon
- 1 small, firm apple chopped into cubes
- 1/2 scoop unsweetened protein powder
- 1 tablespoon ground flaxseed
- 1 cup milk
- 1 cup cubed ice

Method

1. Blend together until the perfect consistency.

Chia Berry

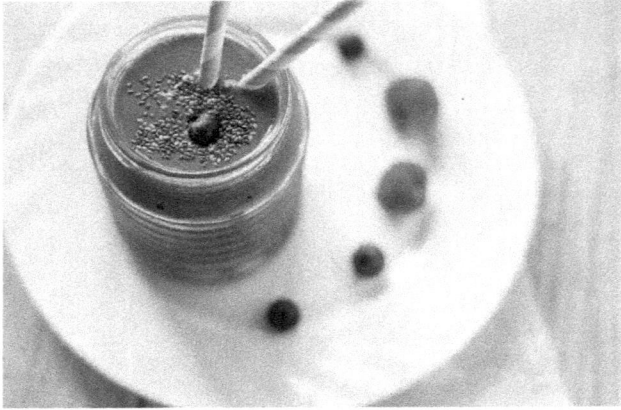

This is a very simple smoothie with a powerful punch. Chia seeds are high in protein and in antioxidants. They also contain Vitamin C which will keep your immune system strong.

The berries provide additional Vitamin C and fiber which will keep you full. This berry delicious smoothie is a fantastic afternoon snack or evening meal. When you want something sweet but are trying to lose weight this smoothie is the perfect choice.

Ingredients

- 1 cup frozen mixed berries or fresh berries of your choice
- 1/2 cup unsweetened pomegranate juice
- 1/2 cup water
- 1/2 tablespoon chia seeds
- 1 cup cubed ice

Method

1. Blend until smooth. Add some chia seeds on the top for garnish if you want.

Bloat Buster

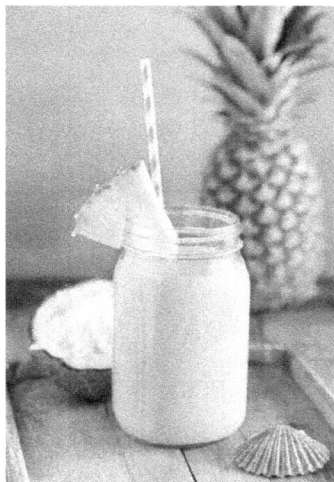

Did you break your diet and have a fancy dinner, pizza, pie or some other indulgence? It's ok. This bloat busting smoothie will flatten your tummy, get rid of that bloat, and get you back on track to lose weight. If you have a tight dress to fit into this smoothie will knock out that water weight so you have a great flat stomach. It's also a delicious snack at any time.

Ingredients

- 1 cup vanilla or plain nonfat Greek yogurt
- 1 tablespoon almond butter or peanut butter
- 1/2 cup frozen or fresh blueberries
- 1/2 cup frozen pineapple or fresh pineapple cut in cubes
- 1 cup kale, chopped fine
- 1 cup coconut water

Method

1. Blend in a blend or mix with a hand blender until smooth.

Classic Apple Cinnamon

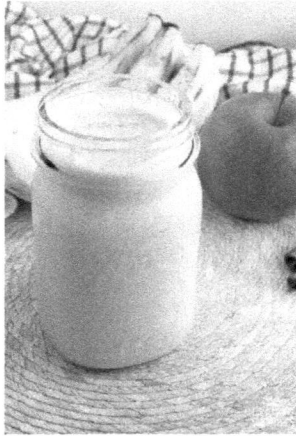

This creamy and delicious apple cinnamon smoothie is breakfast of champions and of Hollywood stars. When you want to drop a few pounds or if you're in a hurry but you still want to eat a breakfast that will keep you full and focused all morning long so that you aren't tempted to grab a doughnut or snack before lunch this is the smoothie you should have. It's a fantastic low-calorie breakfast that will keep you satisfied until lunch.

Ingredients

- ½ cup ground almonds
- 1 red apple, peeled and cut into chunks
- 1 banana, sliced into chunks
- 1 cup vanilla Greek yogurt
- 1/2 cup nonfat milk
- 1 teaspoon cinnamon

Method

1. Blend and enjoy on the go.

Classic Clean Berry

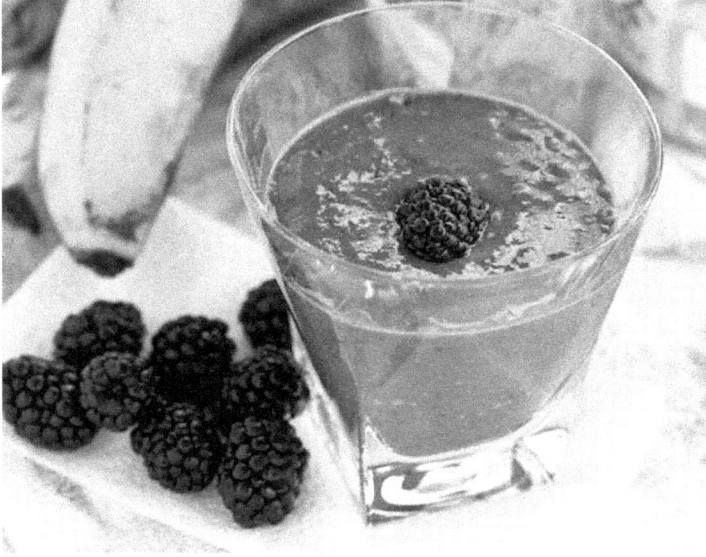

If you're a fan of "clean" eating this smoothie is going to be one that you make often. It's made from "clean" ingredients that you can enjoy anytime when you want a boost of antioxidant power and a protein infusion to keep you from getting hungry. This tasty berry treat is sure to please when you're craving sweets.

Ingredients

- 1 cup almond milk
- 1 scoop chocolate protein powder or vanilla if you prefer.
- 1 banana, cut into chunks
- 1 cup blackberries, fresh or frozen
- 1 cup cubed ice

Method

1. Blend until creamy then enjoy.

Banana Bread

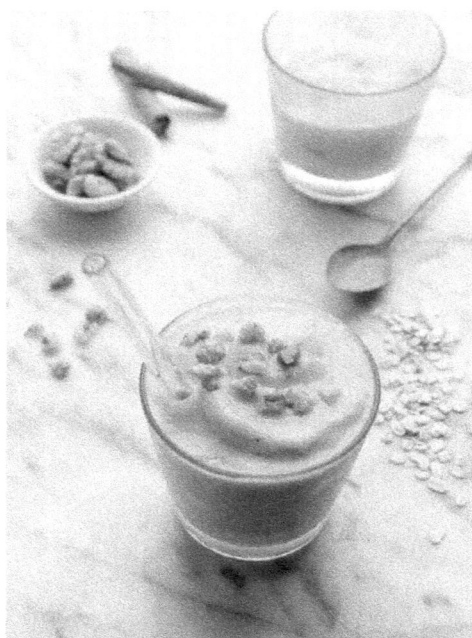

This amazing breakfast smoothie clocks in with more than 34 grams of protein per serving. If you are tempted by sweet morning treats like doughnuts and pastries this delicious smoothie will give you the sweetness and creaminess that you want without all those calories and the high fat of breakfast treats.

Chow down on this delicious smoothie when you feel like you could eat a whole stack of pancakes.

Ingredients

- 1/2 cup low-fat cottage cheese or Greek yogurt
- 1/2 cup vanilla almond milk
- 1/2 medium banana, cut in chunks
- 1 scoop vanilla protein powder

- 2 tablespoons chopped walnuts
- 1/2 teaspoon vanilla extract
- 1 teaspoon cinnamon
- 1/2 teaspoon nutmeg

Method

1. Blend well and enjoy. Top with cinnamon for some extra flavor.

Classic Papaya

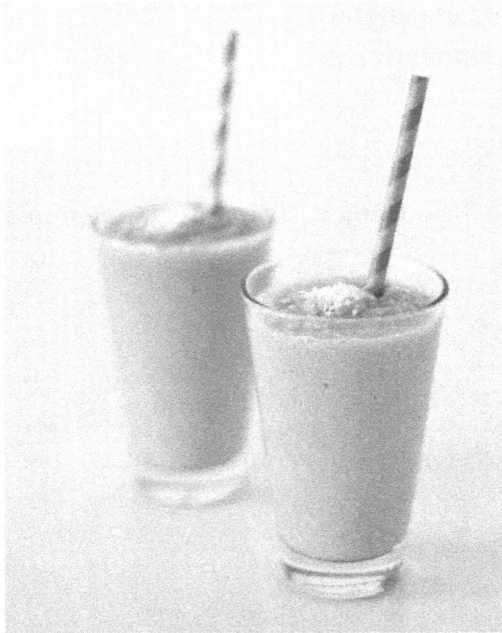

This smoothie is great for fighting bloat and water weight gain. If you need to flush out your system so that you can detox or if you need to lose some water weight fast this fresh and classic smoothie is the perfect choice.

When you first start a weight loss regimen you should make one of these smoothies every day for the first couple of days to help flush fat and toxins from your body.

Ingredients

- 1/2 cup pineapple
- 1/2 cup papaya
- 1 frozen banana
- ½ cup of diced cucumber with the peel on

148

- 1 cup chilled coconut water
- 2 cups spinach, chopped fine
- 1 cup cubed ice

Method

1. Combine all the ingredients and blend.

Peanut Butter Banana

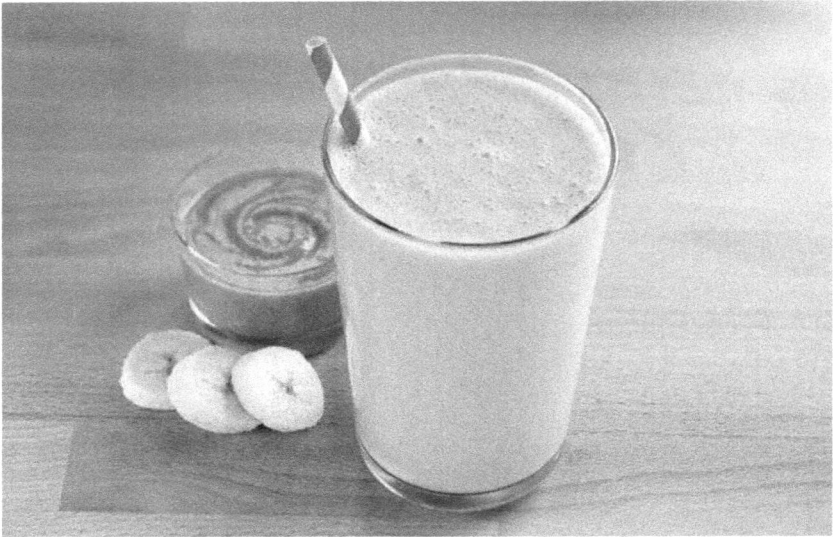

This smoothie is a hearty meal replacement that has the protein and fiber to keep you full. If you know you're going to have a long day or if you know you're going to be too busy to grab lunch or dinner later on this smoothie makes the perfect snack or breakfast.

Ingredients

- 1 banana, chopped up into pieces
- ½ cup of peanut butter, almond bar, or cashew butter
- 1 cup of vanilla almond milk
- 1 cup of cubed ice

Method

1. Blend thoroughly and enjoy.

Chocolate Chocolate Chocolate

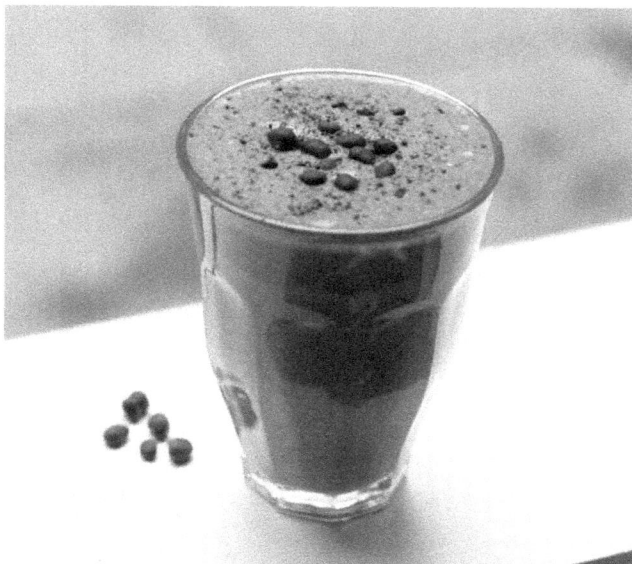

Sometimes even when you are dieting you just have to have some chocolate. And chocolate can be good for you, in moderation. This tasty treat will give you that deep chocolate taste you are craving along with a nice energy shot. It's the perfect snack for the late morning or the late afternoon when you still have a lot to do and you need a sweet snack to keep you going.

Ingredients

- 2 tablespoons of dark chocolate cocoa powder
- 1/2 cup of almond milk
- 1 cup of low-fat vanilla frozen yogurt
- 1 shot of cold espresso

Method

1. Blend together and enjoy.

Summer Watermelon

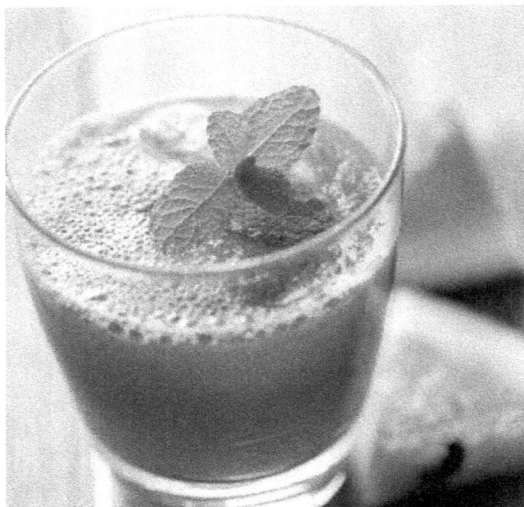

There's nothing better than a watermelon smoothie when the temperature climbs and the sun is beating down. This delicious fruity smoothie is the perfect smoothie to enjoy after a swim, on the beach, or after a hot summer workout. It also can be a refreshing drink at the end of a long day. In fact, you can drink it almost all day long because it is so low in calories yet packed with nutrients.

Ingredients

- 6 cups of seedless watermelon, chopped small
- 1 cup of lemon sherbet
- 1 cup vanilla low fat yogurt
- 1 cup cubed ice

Method

1. Blend together for a perfect summer smoothie. Garnish with a little mint if you want a little refreshing kick.

Classic Blueberry

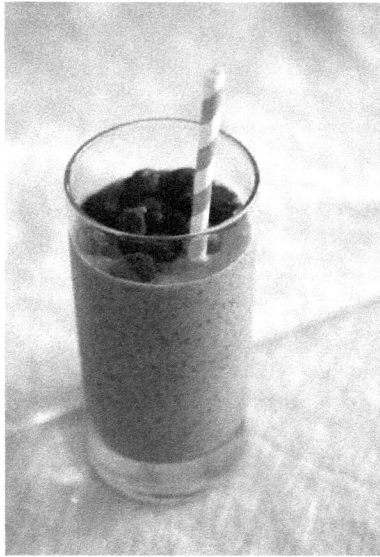

This back to basic smoothie is old school but delicious and brimming with antioxidants. This smoothie will kick your immune system into high gear and give you a great hit of natural energy that will keep you going. This is a perfect snack smoothie that you can share with your kids.

Ingredients

- 1 cup frozen or fresh blueberries
- 1 banana, sliced thin
- 1 cup fat free milk
- 1 cup cubed ice

Method

1. Blend all the ingredients and enjoy. Add some fresh orange juice for a citrus twist.

California Classic

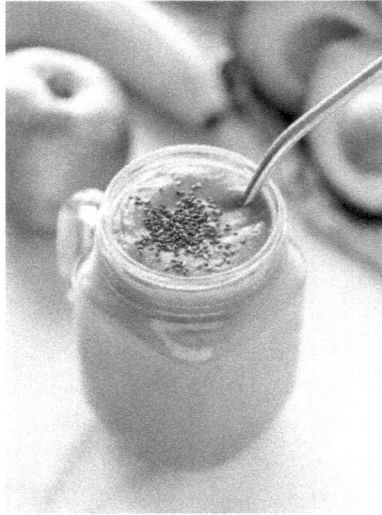

Avocados are one of the healthiest things you can eat. They are full of healthy fats that will make you feel full without a lot of calories. This classic smoothie born in the state of sunshine and healthy food will give you all the green power you need to stay healthy and lose weight.

Ingredients

- 6 ounces of nonfat yogurt
- 1 banana, cut into chunks
- ½ an avocado
- ¼ cup apple juice
- ¾ cup carrot juice
- 1 cup cubed ice

Method

1. Pour into a blender and blend thoroughly.

Sunny Day

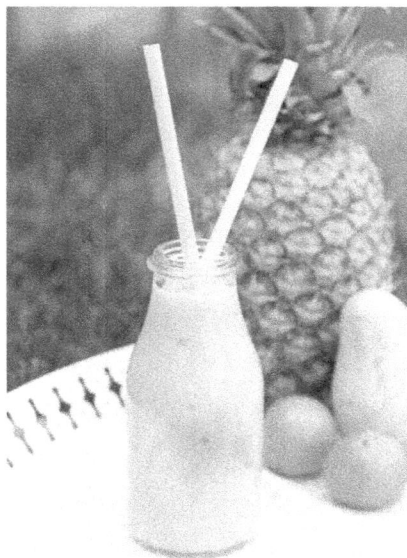

This citrus smoothie is perfect for weight loss. The antioxidants in the citrus fruit will kick start your weight loss and the Vitamin C will boost your immune system so that you will stay healthy even though your body is going through a lot of changes. This is also a great pick me up when it's cold or rainy outside.

Ingredients

- 1 banana, sliced into chunks
- ½ cup fresh orange juice
- 2 small oranges, peeled and separated into segments
- ½ cup pineapple chunks, can be fresh or frozen
- 1 cup mango chunks, can be fresh or frozen

Method

1. Blend and enjoy.

Power Food Pick Me Up

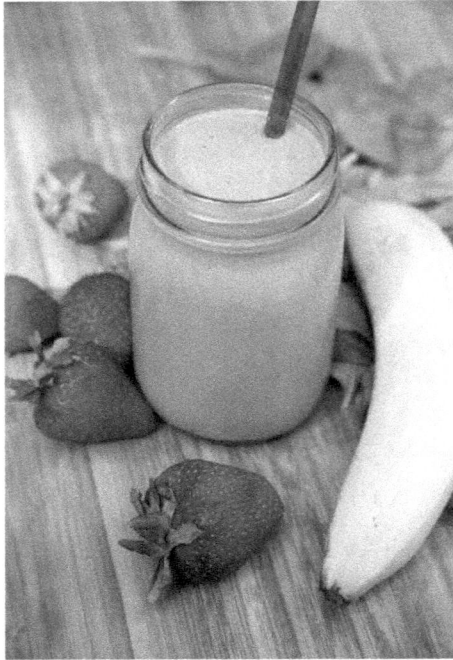

When you need some serious pick up to face a really long day, a marathon workout, or another huge task this is the smoothie to choose.

It is full of green power and antioxidants from fresh fruit that will supercharge your body and give you energy to burn. This smoothie will give you enough energy to last all day if necessary and it tastes great.

Ingredients

- 2 bananas cut into chunks
- 1 cup of fresh or frozen spinach, chopped small
- ¼ cup fresh or frozen strawberries, sliced

- 2 tablespoons of ground flaxseed
- 1 small apple, peeled and chopped
- 1 cup vanilla almond milk
- 1 cup of cubed ice

Method

1. Blend thoroughly and drink.

Key Lime Pie

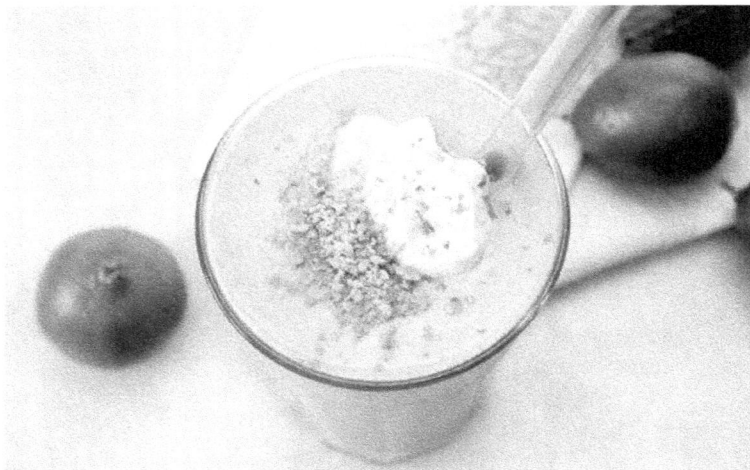

This deliciously tangy and refreshing smoothie brings to mind summer days and cooling key lime treats but without the calories of an actual key lime pie. When you are craving sweets or just want to beat the heat, this smoothie is a fabulous snack or quick breakfast if you are running out the door.

Ingredients

- 1 cup of vanilla frozen yogurt
- ½ cup of fresh key lime or lime juice
- ½ cup milk
- 1 tablespoon of vanilla coffee creamer
- ½ tablespoon of vanilla extract
- 1 graham cracker, crumbled

Method

1. Blend everything but the graham cracker. Sprinkle that on top and enjoy.

Cleansing

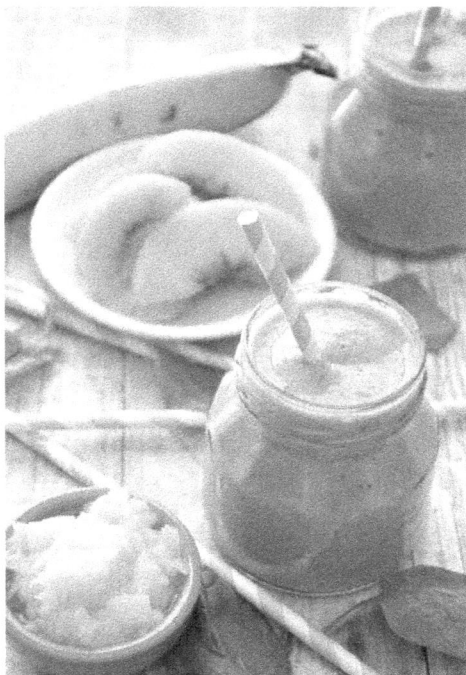

Part of losing weight is cleaning your body. You need to clean out all the fat and waste that your body is shedding so that you be healthy and look slimmer.

Water weight, bloat and other problems all stem from impurities in the body. This powerful smoothie will get rid of those wastes, end the bloat, and help you lose weight and stay healthy.

Ingredients

- 1 banana, chopped into small pieces
- 1 cup pineapple chunks, fresh or frozen
- ½ cup almond milk or rice milk
- 1 small peach, chopped into pieces

- ½ cup plain Greek yogurt
- 1 cup of spinach, fresh or frozen, chopped small
- 1 cup of cubed ice

Method

1. Blend well and enjoy.

Strawberry Mango Madness

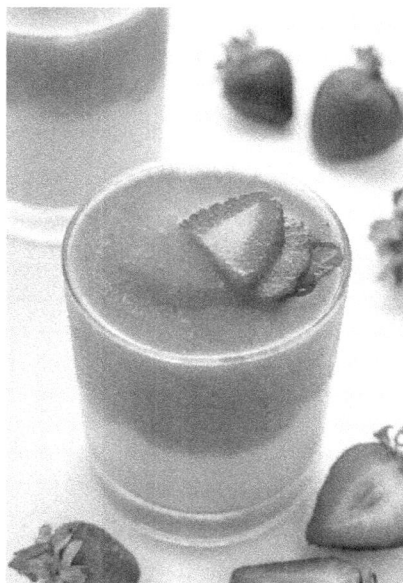

This beautiful smoothie is a feast for the eyes as well for the mouth. It's pretty bright colors and delicious lush fruit taste make it great for a snack but hearty enough to be a wonderful summer breakfast. If you want to make a healthy and sweet dessert that will satisfy those after dinner cravings this is the smoothie for you.

Ingredients

- 2 large bananas, cut into chunks
- 1 cup mango chunks, fresh or frozen
- ½ cup of orange juice
- ¼ cup of fresh or frozen strawberries, sliced
- ½ cup strawberry Greek yogurt
- ¼ cup of milk
- ¼ cup granola

Method

1. For this smoothie, you are going to make layers. So first blend the bananas, mango and orange juice.

2. Pour that on the bottom of the glass. Then layer the granola on top of that.

3. When that is done blend the strawberries, Greek yogurt and milk. Layer that on top of the granola.

Peanut Butter Cup

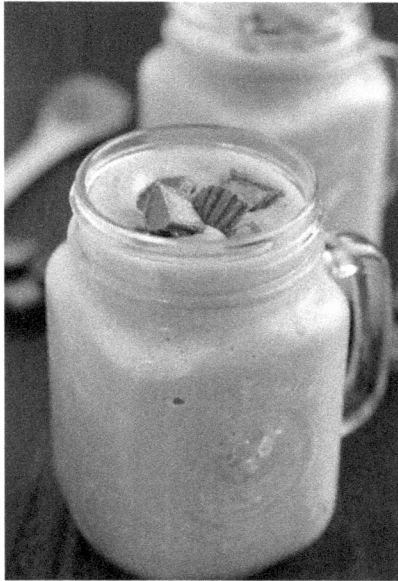

This simple but tasty smoothie tastes like your favorite candy bar but has less than half the calories of a candy bar. It also has more than 28 grams of super healthy protein. This is a great smoothie to make before you work out or for an afternoon or evening snack.

Ingredients

- 6 ounces of vanilla Greek yogurt
- ½ cup of fat free milk or almond milk
- ¼ cup natural peanut butter, chunky or plain
- 1 tablespoon dark cocoa powder
- 1 cup of cubed ice

Method

1. Blend thoroughly and enjoy.

Funfetti

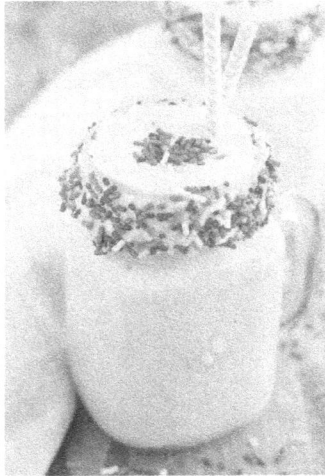

This smoothie is the perfect treat for birthdays or other events when everyone else is eating cake but you are trying to lose weight. Stick with your smoothies and stay on track with this healthy alternative to cake. It's delicious and tastes like cake without all the fat and the high calories.

Ingredients

- 2 large bananas cut into chunks and frozen
- ½ cup vanilla almond milk
- ½ cup vanilla Greek yogurt
- ½ teaspoon of vanilla extract
- 1 tablespoon of rainbow sprinkles

Method

1. Blend all the ingredients together except the sprinkles. When the smoothie is nice and frothy put the sprinkles on the top to make it more festive and add a little touch of sweetness.

Orange Creamsicle

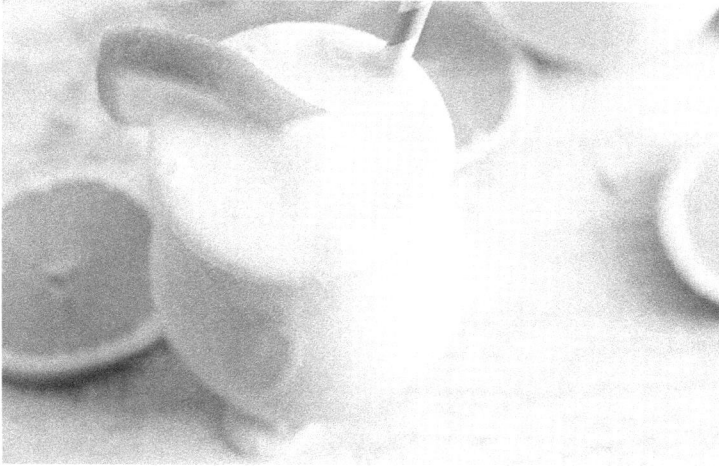

This light and sweet treat tastes like a summer day. It's a fantastic alternative to frozen ice cream treats in the summer and it's so healthy you can have it for breakfast. If you want to cool off and enjoy summer sweets without all the calories this creamy cool citrus treat is the best choice.

Ingredients

- 1 banana, cut into chunks and frozen
- 2 teaspoons of vanilla extract
- ¼ cup fresh orange juice
- ¾ cup of vanilla Greek yogurt
- 1 orange, peeled and cut into chunks
- 1 teaspoon of orange zest

Method

1. Combine all the ingredients and whip in the blender, expect the orange zest. Sprinkle that on top as a great garnish.

PB&J

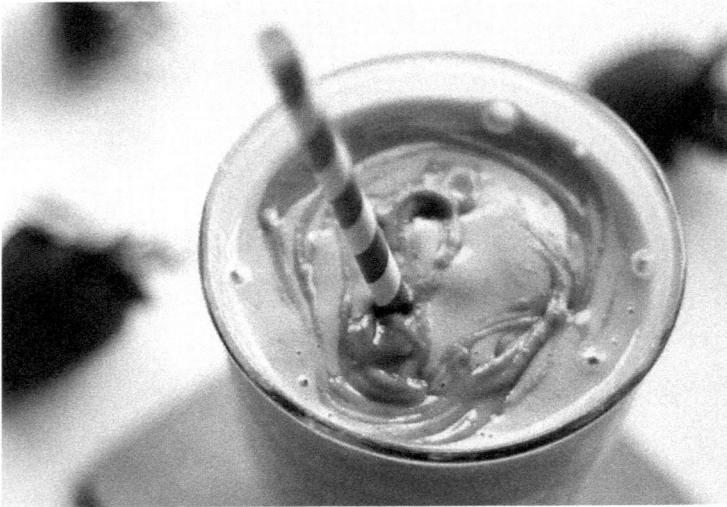

Everyone loves a good PB&J but now you can enjoy yours without the calories and the added sugar. This smoothie is super filling and it's a great meal replacement. If you have to skip lunch or you want to cut calories for dinner this is a super smoothie to have because it will keep you full for hours.

Ingredients

- 1 banana, cut into chunks
- ½ cup of strawberry Greek yogurt
- 2 tablespoons of peanut butter, either chunky or smooth
- ¾ cup of milk
- 1 cup of strawberries, fresh or frozen but sliced thin

Method

1. Blend everything together. It will be thick. If it's too thick for you add more milk.

Skinny Almond

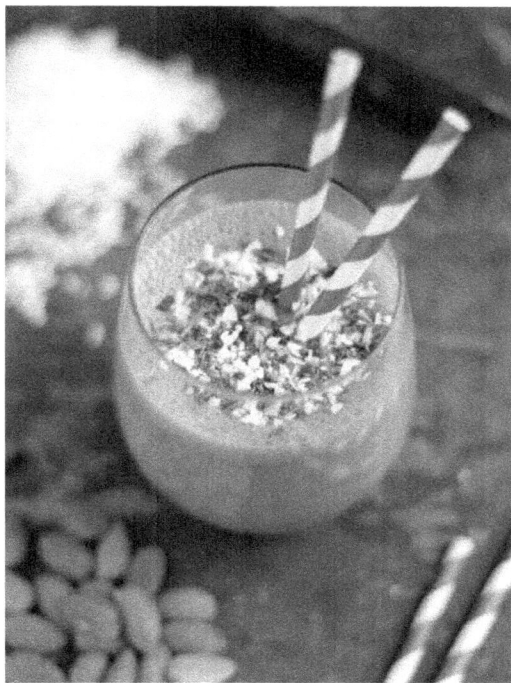

If you love almond, chocolate and coconut candy bars this smoothie is going to be your favorite treat.

It tastes as good as a candy bar but is so much healthier. It will give you the energy that you need to power through a workout or go home and take care of your family after working all day. This smoothie tastes like a sweet treat but really, it's good for you.

Ingredients

- 2 bananas, sliced and frozen
- 1 tablespoon of dark cocoa powder
- 2/3 cup almond milk
- ½ cup plain Greek yogurt

- ½ teaspoon of coconut extract
- ½ teaspoon of almond extract
- 2 tablespoons of chopped almonds

Method

1. Combine everything and blend until mixed thoroughly.

Mint Chocolate

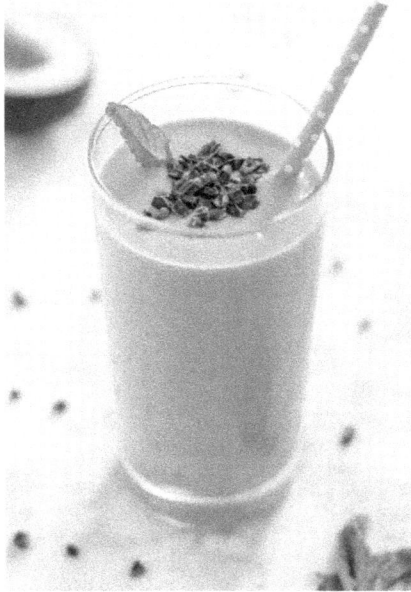

This is a decadent tasting smoothie that won't blow your weight loss. When you have to have a chocolate treat you can indulge with this smoothie that actually is good for you but the rich chocolate taste that you're craving. The fresh mint adds a nice brightness to the chocolate and makes this smoothie refreshing as well as delicious.

Ingredients

- 3 ripe bananas, frozen
- 3 tablespoons of dark cocoa powder
- ½ cup of milk
- 1 cup of vanilla Greek yogurt
- ¼ teaspoon peppermint extract
- 2-4 fresh mint leaves

Method

1. Combine everything but the mint leaves in the blend and blend on high. Add the mint leaves as a garnish when serving.

Pumpkin Pie

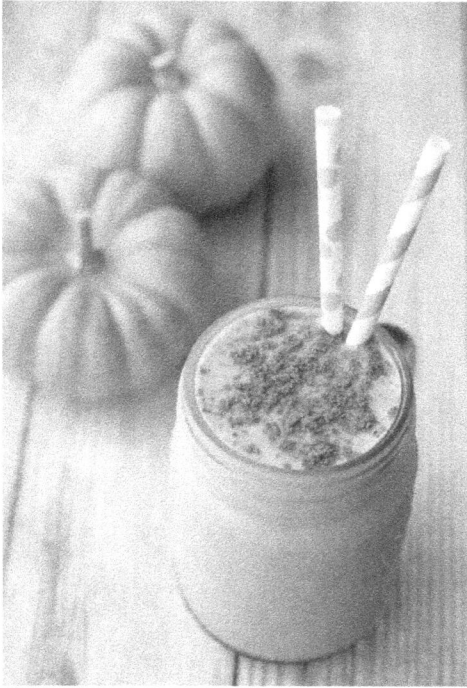

Love fall pumpkin drinks and treats but don't want the added calories and sugar? This healthy version of your favorite fall treats will give you all that pumpkin spice flavor that you love without all the stuff you don't want. This will become your go-to treat for fall.

When your friends are all complaining about gaining that holiday weight you can smile knowing you had your pumpkin pie and lost weight too.

Ingredients

- 1 ½ cups of cold coffee
- 1 ¼ cups of vanilla almond milk
- 1 banana, cut into pieces

- ½ cup of pumpkin puree
- 3 tablespoons of pure maple syrup or honey
- 2 tablespoons of pumpkin pie spice

Method

1. Whip everything together in a blender and enjoy.

Purple Power Food

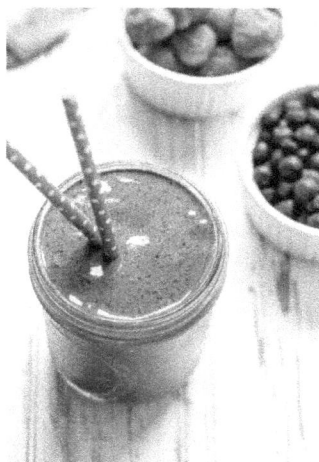

This smoothie is jam packed with berry goodness. It has enough antioxidants to help your skin and your body stay heathy. It also has more than 28 essential nutrients that you need to lose weight and stay healthy. On top of that it has enough protein and rich taste to keep you feeling full for hours. This is truly a power drink that is the perfect way to start the morning or the perfect way to end the day.

Ingredients

- ½ cup fresh or frozen raspberries
- ½ cup fresh or frozen blueberries
- ½ cup coconut water
- ½ cup blueberry Greek yogurt
- 1 tablespoon of honey
- 1 cup cubed ice

Method

1. Blend together and enjoy the purple power.

Quick Berry

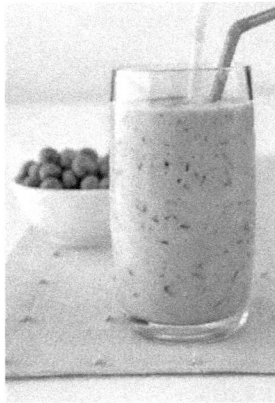

Sometimes you really need to grab something to fill you up but you just don't have a lot of time. This happens a lot in the morning, especially to people who have a hard time getting up on time. If you need a tried and true quick and delicious smoothie that you can make in under five minutes as you are rushing out the door this is the best smoothie you can make in that time frame. It's full of healthy berries and more than 30 grams of protein to keep you full until you can grab your next meal.

Ingredients

- 6 ounces of blueberry Greek yogurt
- 1 cup of frozen or fresh blueberries
- 1 scoop vanilla protein powder
- ½ cubed ice
- 1 cup milk or water

Method

1. Blend everything together and you will be on your way in minutes.

Tropical Green

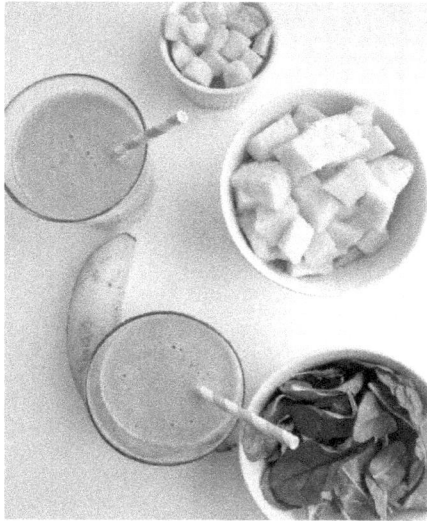

This citrus-based smoothie tastes like a tropical cocktail but has all the nutrition you need to get through the day without being hungry. When you want a quick boost of energy or a refreshing drink that will fill you up this is the best smoothie to choose. Best of all is that it has less than 200 calories per serving.

Ingredients

- 2 cups fresh spinach, cut small or frozen spinach
- 1 cup vanilla almond milk
- 1 banana chopped into pieces and frozen
- 1 cup chopped fresh or frozen mango
- 1 cup chopped fresh or frozen pineapple
- 1 cup of cubed ice

Method

1. Blend everything together and drink.

Chocolate Silk

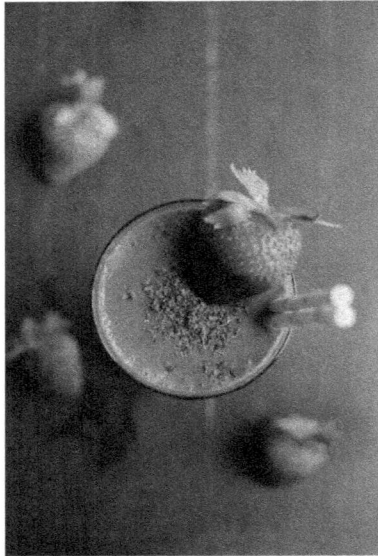

There's nothing more decadent than chocolate silk pie. But this smoothie gives you the rich and creamy taste of chocolate silk pie in a low calorie and protein packed drink that you can take anywhere. Keep your weight loss on track but satisfy those chocolate cravings with this low-calorie substitute for chocolate pie.

Ingredients

- 1 cup frozen or fresh strawberries, sliced
- ¼ cup dark cocoa powder
- 1 cup vanilla almond milk
- 1 cup of cubed ice
- 1 banana, cut into small pieces

Method

1. Blend until thoroughly mixed and enjoy.

Carrot Orange

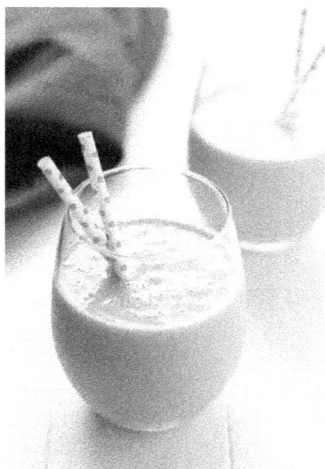

This unique smoothie sweet and citrusy but it is filled with some of the most powerful nutrients you can get in a glass. The unique taste is rich and deep and makes a fantastic breakfast smoothie. This is also a great drink to have after a workout when you need to replenish your electrolytes and nourish your muscles.

Ingredients

- ½ cup plain Greek yogurt
- ¼ cup lime juice
- 1/2 cup carrot juice
- 1/2 cup orange juice
- 3/4 cup frozen mango
- 3/4 cup frozen pineapple
- 1 cup cubed ice

Method

1. Whip and enjoy.

End of the Day Treat

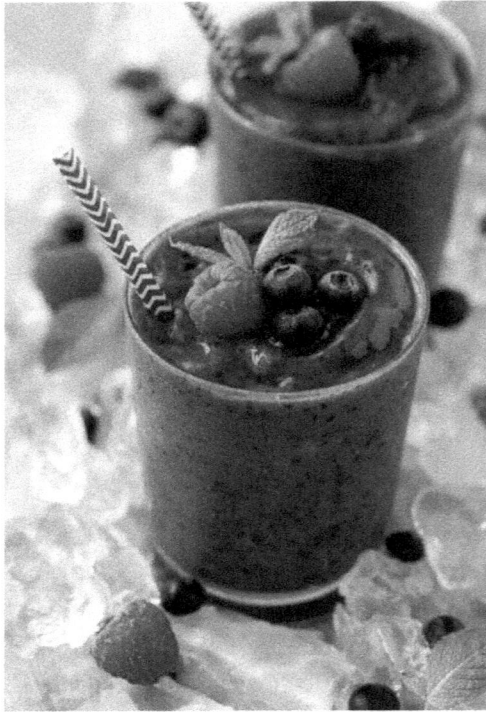

When the day is done and you want a sweet treat this smoothie will help you stay away from the cookies, cake and other junk food that made you gain weight in the first place.

When you are trying to lose weight but you are having fierce cravings for a night time treat or when you need a sweet pick me up in the late afternoon to get through the day this smoothie is the perfect choice.

Ingredients

- 1 cup fresh or frozen raspberries
- 1 cup fresh or frozen blackberries

- ½ cup instant oats
- 1 cup milk
- 1 ripe banana, fresh or frozen
- 1 tablespoon of almond butter
- 2 tablespoons of granola

Method

1. Whip the berries, the oats, the banana and the milk together. Pour into a cup or bowl. Top with the granola and the almond butter.

Cucumber Melon

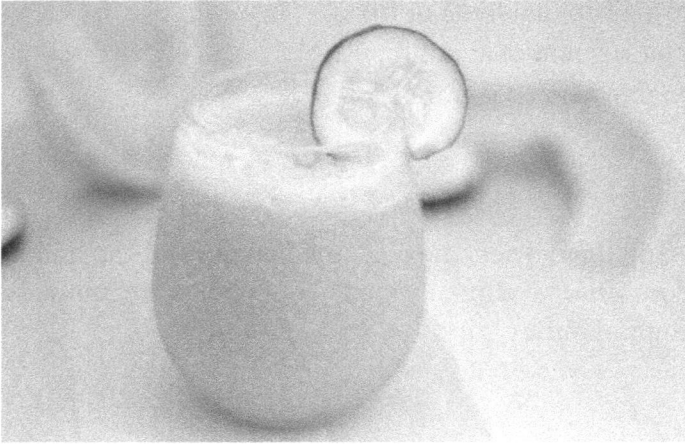

This is a super simple but super delicious smoothie that is perfect for hot summer days. Whether you want a cool and refreshing treat or a light and nutrient packed breakfast this deliciously cool smoothie has it.

This is also a great smoothie to serve by the pool at summer gatherings. Kids love it and it will keep them hydrated throughout the long summer days.

Ingredients

- 1 cup water
- ½ honeydew melon, cubed
- 1 small cucumber peeled, seeded and sliced
- 1 cup cubed or shaved ice

Method

1. Blend and serve. Garnish with a slice of cucumber if you want to.

Cantaloupe Melon Madness

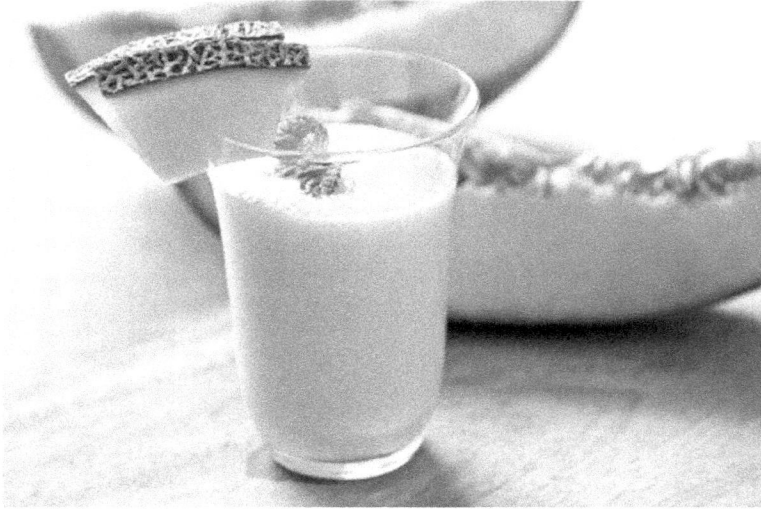

This is another really simple melon smoothie that is fantastic for breakfast or as a dessert. Melons are packed with water, which will help you flush out fat and toxins from your system. They are also filled with more than 28 nutrients that your body needs to stay fit and healthy. So, make this cantaloupe classic all summer long whenever you need a sweet and juicy treat.

Ingredients

- 1 cantaloupe, scooped out and chopped into small cubes
- 1 cup of Greek yogurt
- 1 cup of cubed ice
- 1 cup of water
- 2 tablespoons of honey

Method

1. Combine in a blender and whip until frothy.

Tropical Protein

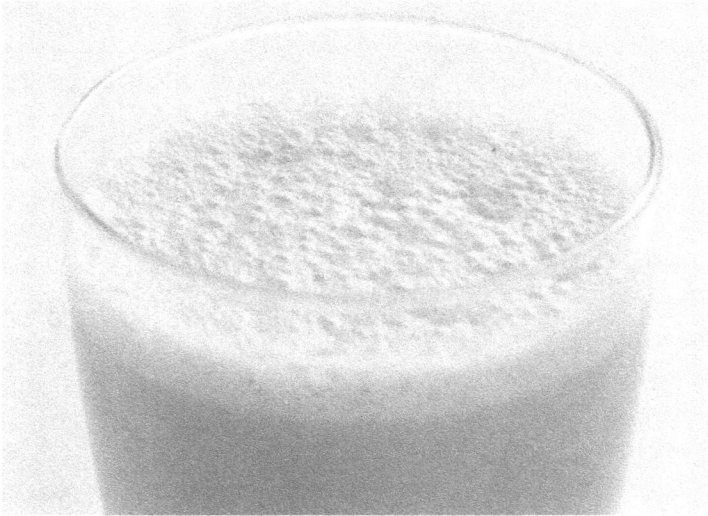

This coconut rich smoothie is great for anyone who loves the exotic taste of coconut. It's packed with the healthy lean protein that you need to lose weight. The protein powder in the smoothie will keep you full for hours between meals so that you won't be tempted to snack. Protein powder also gives your muscles the nutrients they need to repair small tears and other injuries that can come from working out.

Ingredients

- 1 scoop vanilla protein powder
- 1 cup frozen mixed tropical fruit
- 1 cup vanilla almond milk
- ½ teaspoon of coconut extract

Method

1. Blend until smooth then drink.

Back to Basics

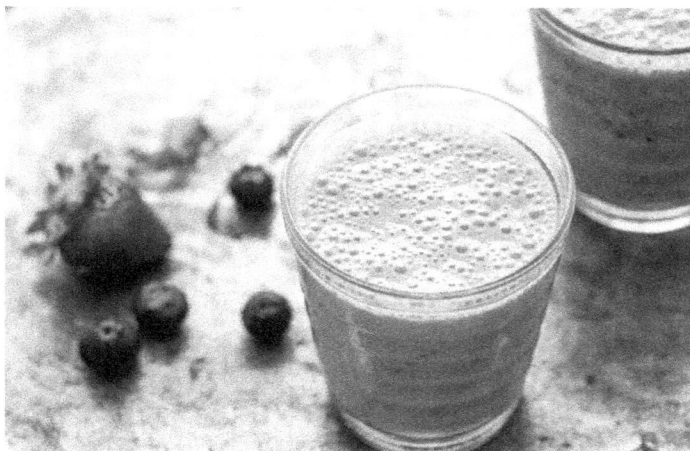

This simple smoothie is tasty, filled with nutrition and requires no special ingredients. You can make it easily with whatever you have in the pantry.

When you need to whip up a quick no-frills smoothie because you are pressed for time or because you just don't want to go to the store for special ingredients this is the smoothie to choose. Adjust the ingredients to whatever you have on hand.

Ingredients

- 1 banana, frozen or fresh
- 1 cup blueberries
- 1 cup strawberries
- 1 cup milk or vanilla yogurt

Method

1. Blend and enjoy. Feel free to use whatever you have on hand instead of the fruit listed.

Blueberry Blast

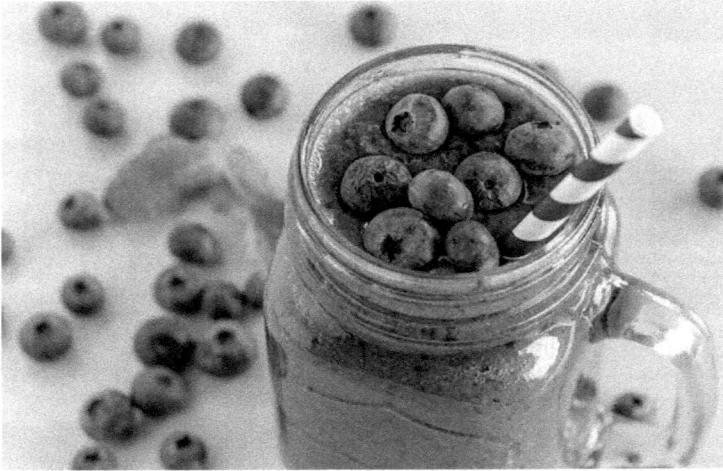

This smoothie contains a blast of Vitamin C and antioxidants that will boost your immune system and help you fight off any germs that are attacking. Sometimes when you diet to lose weight you get run down and your immune system doesn't function the way it should. This Blueberry Blast smoothie should fix you right up and get you back to feeling great in no time.

Ingredients

- 1 cup fresh or frozen blueberries
- 1 cup pomegranate juice
- ½ cup orange juice
- 1 cup cubed or crushed ice
- 1 packet of Vitamin C crystals
- 1 banana

Method

1. Blend well and enjoy.

Pina Colada

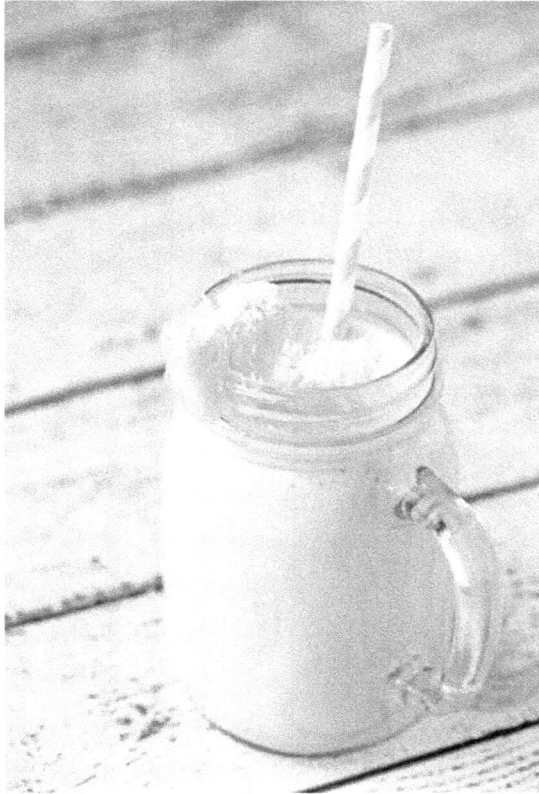

Pina Colada is the perfect drink for summer and this Pina Colada smoothie is the perfect summer breakfast. It also can be a nice dessert. As a breakfast replacement, this smoothie provides enough protein to keep you going until lunch along with the smooth creamy taste that people enjoy in the morning.

Ingredients

- ½ cup instant oats
- 1 cup coconut milk
- 1 cup vanilla or plain yogurt

- 1 cup crushed pineapple
- 1 tablespoon honey or agave
- ¼ cup of toasted coconut for garnish
- 1 cup crushed or cubed ice

Method

1. Combine all the ingredients expect the toasted coconut and blend. Garnish with the toasted coconut.

Green Tea

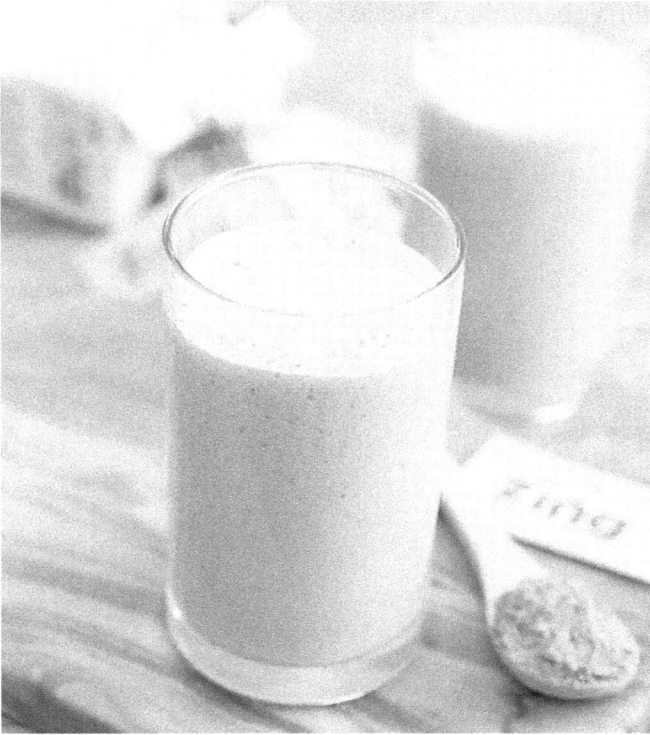

Green tea is one of the healthiest things that you can drink. In addition to having nutrients and antioxidants green tea has been proven to help with weight loss. A green tea smoothie is a fantastic choice when you are trying to lose weight. This tasty smoothie will make you forget that it's actually really healthy for you because it's sweet and tastes so rich and delicious.

Ingredients

- 1 cup frozen or fresh white seedless grapes
- 1 cup of fresh or frozen spinach
- 1 1/2 cups strong green tea, cooled

- 1 avocado
- 2 teaspoons honey
- 1 cup cubed or crushed ice

Method

1. Blend until frothy then enjoy.

Watermelon Mint Mojito

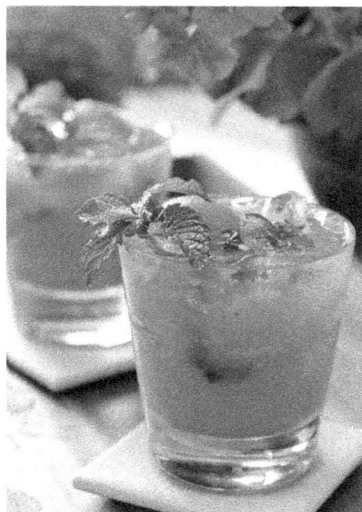

If you're tired of the same old smoothies and you want to try something different and delicious this is the smoothie for you. It's so refreshing and yet so healthy. Watermelon is full of healthy water to help you lose weight and it also contains Lycopene and antioxidants. The light and refreshing smoothie is great for hot summer days or nights.

Ingredients

- 2 cups diced watermelon
- ½ cup lime juice
- 1 cup water
- 8-10 fresh mint leaves, chopped
- 1 cup crushed ice

Method

1. Blend together and drink frosty cold.

Purple Dragon

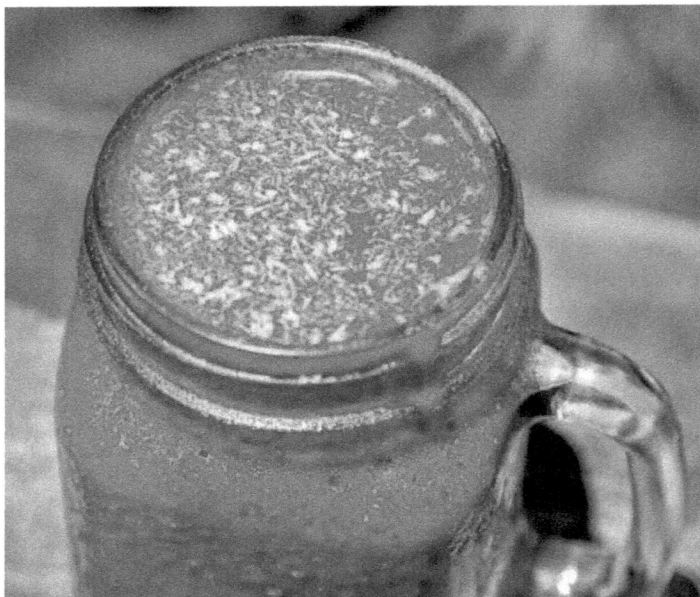

This exotic smoothie is filled with all kinds of delicious and healthy fruits and vegetables. Combined they deliver more than 30 of the essential vitamins and minerals that you need to lose weight and be healthy.

Plus, they provide the protein and fiber you need to stay full and satisfied. Just one of these special smoothies packs a powerful nutritional punch and an amazing taste that you will love.

Ingredients

- 8 ounces of almond milk
- 2 cups of baby spinach, chopped
- 1 banana cut into chunks and frozen
- ½ cup frozen or fresh dragon fruit
- ½ cup frozen blueberries

- ¼ cup ground almonds
- 2 Medjool dates
- 1 tablespoon Acai powder
- 1 tablespoon Chia seeds
- 2 tablespoons of shredded coconut for garnish

Method

1. Combine all the ingredients in a powerful blender that can break up frozen fruit. Garnish with the shredded coconut and more Chia seeds if you want.

Chocolate Almond Oatmeal

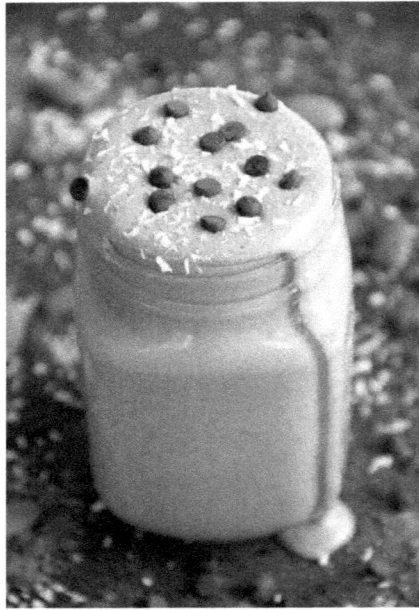

This sweet and hearty breakfast smoothie is the perfect choice when you want a healthy and filling breakfast in a hurry. Maybe you are rushing off to work, maybe you are rushing to get the kids to school or maybe you are rushing to go workout. But whatever you're doing means you're in a hurry and need a good breakfast.

This is the smoothie to choose when that happens. Rich chocolate and healthy oatmeal make a smoothie that tastes great but will help you lose weight too.

Ingredients

- 1 cup instant oats
- 1 cup of chocolate almond milk
- 1 large banana, cut into chunks

- ½ cup ground almonds
- 1 cup of cubed or crushed ice

Method

1. Blend together and enjoy.

I hope you have learned something from this book so far and would greatly appreciate it if you could leave an honest review on Amazon.com.

16 Special Summer Juices That Are Quick & Easy to Make!

Summer is a time that everyone looks forward to. They are excited for the warm days that seem to last so much longer than normal, yet not long enough.

The time that they get to hang out with family and friends and do the things that they love, or at least get things done outside around the house.

But when you are done with all of that hard work, or have spent a long day outside in the warm weather, there's nothing tastier than a good, cold drink.

Instead of just drinking water or running out of ideas on what to serve at your next party, check out these delicious recipes ahead.

Give a few a try and enjoy the healthy tastes that summer has to offer.

Sunrise Margarita

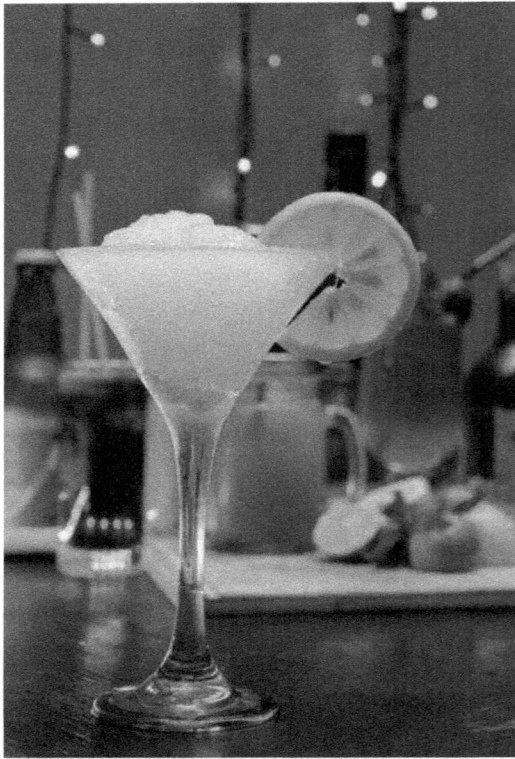

This is such an easy and great to look at cocktail that will give you all of the flavors to remind you of summer, no matter what time of year it is. Add some red sugar to the rim of your cup to get a great fiery look that is all its own.

Ingredients

- Red sugar
- 1 wedge of lime
- 2 c. orange liqueur
- 1 ½ c. lime juice
- 2 c. tequila

- 2 c. orange juice
- 1 c. powdered sugar
- Grenadine syrup
- Orange slices
- Ice cubes

Method

1. To start this recipe, place some sugar onto a plate and have it all spread out. Rub the rims of your glasses with a lime wedge before dipping into the sugar and getting all coated. Set to the side.

2. Bring out a big pitcher and combine the sugar, lime juice, tequila, and triple Sec. Stir so that the sugar dissolves and then stir the orange juice. Chill in the fridge until you are ready to serve.

3. Place the ice cubes into your prepared glasses before pouring in the juice mixture and adding 2 sprits of the grenadine syrup. Garnish with the slices of orange if you would like before serving.

The flavors that come in the glass can give you a bright colorful look that is fun for the beach or just relaxing on your porch. Many people find that it is nice for their BBQ's as well. If you need a non-alcoholic beverage, you can remove the tequila and still get a great taste.

June Bug

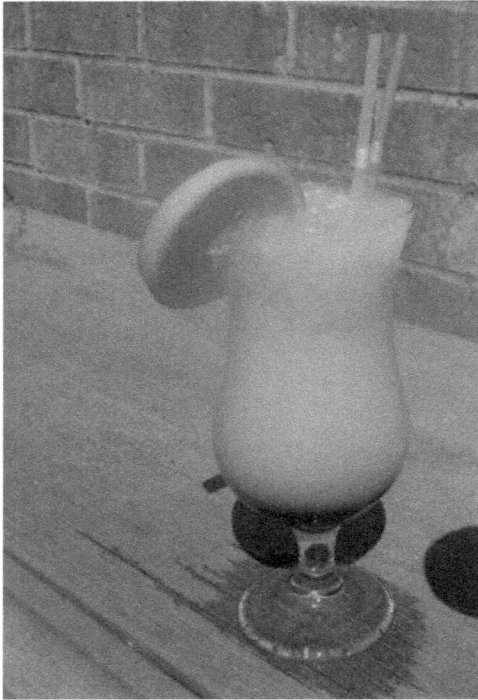

Not every drink for the summer needs to be filled with alcohol and this is a great example. It has some bubblies and some sugar sweetness to fill any hearts' desire and can be enjoyed by kids and adults alike.

Ingredients

- 4 Tbsp. grenadine
- 3 c. ginger ale
- 3 scoops orange sherbet
- 4 Tbsp. orange juice

Method

1. To begin this recipe, blend the sherbet, orange juice, and grenadine together until they are nice and smooth.

2. Pour this into some cocktail glasses that have some ice in them and then enjoy.

If you are serving this at a kids' party or just to your children in the summer, leave the recipe as it is. On the other hand, you can also make this drink more adult friendly by adding in a little bit of white rum.

Cucumber Sangria

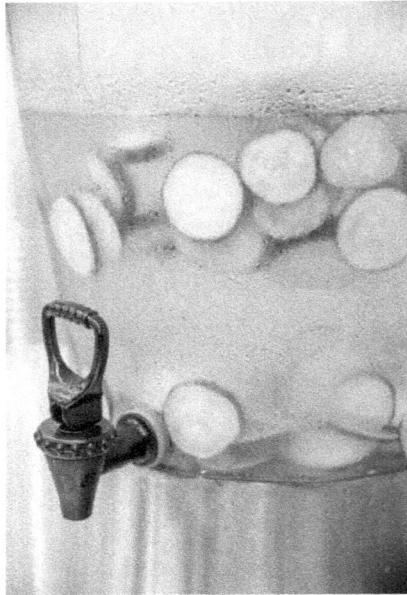

Nothing can cool you down on a hot summers' day than some fresh cucumbers. This drink is a great way to get them in so you can stay refreshed while still getting in your healthy vegetable nutrition. What could be better than that?

Ingredients

- 1 sliced seedless cucumber
- 1 honeydew melon
- 1 sliced lime
- ¼ c. lime juice
- 12 mint leaves, fresh
- ¼ c. honey
- 1 liter chilled carbonated water
- 1 bottle dry white wine

Method

1. To begin this recipe, cut the melon up so that it is in half. Remove and then get rid of the rind and the seeds so that you just have the fruit left. Cut up the rest of the melon so that you have slices.

2. Bring out the pitcher that you have and combine the mint leaves, lime slices, cucumber, and melon inside and set to the side.

3. Take out a bowl and stir together both the honey and the lime juice until they are well combined. Pour over the mixture in the pitcher before adding the wine and stirring a bit. Cover the pitcher and let this drink chill for a minimum of 2 hours.

4. When you are ready to serve, add in the carbonated water of your choice. Ladle this into glasses and then serve.

This mixture is going to make quite a bit of the drink. If you find that you do not have enough room in your fridge for the whole drink, split it up into smaller containers to use some now and some later.

Blackberry Lemonade

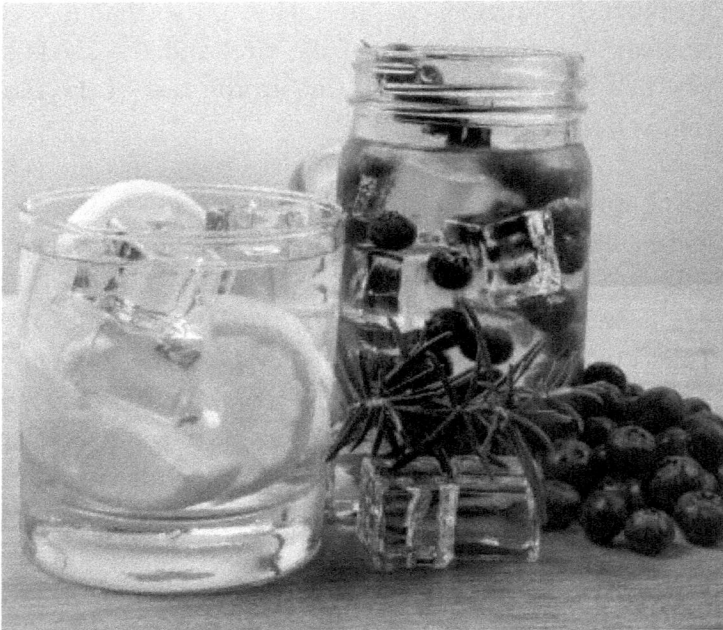

Fruity drinks are the favorites in summer. They taste so good and can add so much refreshment that it can be really difficult to put them down. This one is especially popular and you can make it either with or without the alcohol for your needs.

Ingredients

- 1 ½ Tbsp. lemon juice
- ¼ c. bourbon
- 1/3 c. chilled sparkling lemonade
- 13 oz. blackberries
- ¾ c. water
- ¼ c. sugar
- 1 ½ Tbsp. rosemary

Method

1. The first thing that you should work on is the syrup for the drink. To do this, take out a saucepan and combine the sugar, water, rosemary, and blackberries. Bring this to a boil before reducing the heat and letting this simmer for about 25 minutes.

2. After this time, you can mash up the blackberries and then take the pan from the heat. Allow to cool down before straining through a strainer and into a jar that has been cleaned. Try to get as much liquid out as possible. You can use it to make the drink right away or store for a week.

3. When you are ready to make the drink, bring out a cocktail shaker. Combine the ice, a few tablespoons of the syrup you made, lemon juice, and bourbon.

4. Shake this for around 30 seconds in order to mix and chill the ingredients. Strain this into some glasses that are filled with ice.

5. Top the mixture with some sparkling lemonade and then garnish with a few blackberries if you would like.

If you want to save some time you can combine the lemonade, lemon juice, and bourbon into a glass with some ice and then pour the syrup in to get the colors how you would like.

It is also possible to make a big batch of this drink if you would like to have it for a party. To do this add in a whole recipe of the syrup with 2/3 cups of the lemon juice, and 3 cups bourbon. Add in 4 cups of the lemonade and garnish with the blackberries. This will make 12 servings.

Peach Punch

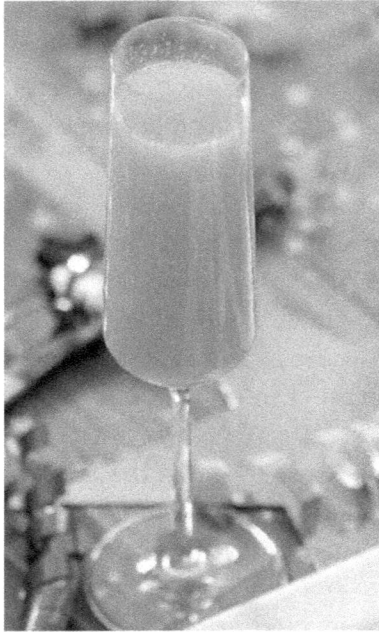

Summer is the time to meet up with friends and family and you never know when someone is going to stop by. This peachy mixture is perfect for throwing into the freezer and pulling out whenever someone shows up unexpectedly.

Ingredients

- 1 ½ c. sugar
- 3 c. water
- 1 can peaches in syrup, sliced
- 1 pkg. gelatin, peach flavored
- ½ c. lemon juice
- 4 cans peach nectar
- 8 bottles ginger ale

Method

1. Take out a pan and combine the gelatin, sugar, and water. Stir and bring to a boil until the sugar and the gelatin until they are dissolved.

2. Next you can bring out a blender and place the peaches inside. Cover the blender and blend these until they become smooth.

3. Now you need a really big bowl and combine the lemon juice, peach nectar, pureed peaches, and gelatin mixture together.

4. Divide up the peach mixture between 4 containers which are a quart each. Cover and let this freeze until it is firm. You can leave in there for 3 months if you would like to have it ready whenever anyone comes.

5. When you are ready to serve, take one of the containers out of the freezer and let it set at a room temperature for an hour.

6. After this time, break it into chunks using a fork and then place inside a jug or a punch bowl. Stir in 2 of the ginger ale bottles for each of the containers you use and then mix so it becomes a slushy. Serve right away.

This is a recipe that is pretty big because it is meant for a storage to use over time. If you would like to use a smaller amount, just halve or quarter the recipe and then make the mixture after freezing just for the night. You can also make the mixture bigger if needed for a large party.

Watermelon Daiquiri

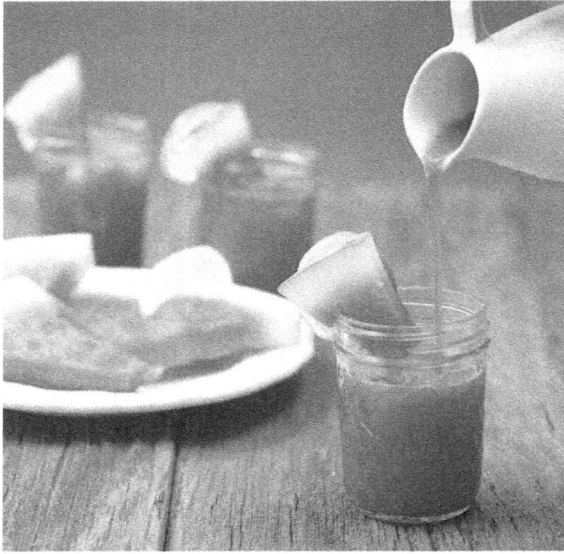

Nothing says summer better than a little bit of watermelon and this drink is going to have you wishing that the beautiful weather never goes away. Shake up the summer a bit with this naturally sweet juice that has a bit of crispness added with the punch of flavor that comes with the basil and rum add to it. Take a taste and see how great summer can be.

Ingredients

- 6 cubes of watermelon
- ¼ c. light rum
- 4 basil leaves
- 1 ½ Tbsp. syrup
- 2 Tbsp. lime juice
- ¼ c. water
- ¼ c. sugar

Method

1. To begin this recipe, you will need to make the syrup. TO do this you should bring out a pan and combine the water and the sugar. Bring this to a light boil, stirring the whole time in order to let the sugar dissolve. Cool this down and let chill for an hour before you use it.

2. Once the syrup is done, take out a cocktail shaker. Combine together the basil and the watermelon and muddle so the watermelon becomes juiced.

3. At this time, add in the ice, simple syrup you made, lime juice, and rum. Shake some more to get it chilled, which will take around 40 seconds.

4. Double strain this into some glasses filled with ice. Garnish with a little extra watermelon and then serve this drink right away.

It is easy to make this into a bigger batch if you would need to serve a larger group. Just make sure to double or triple the ingredients to get the amount that you want. Everyone at the party is going to enjoy the refreshing taste of the drink and you will be the talk of the party.

Pisco Sour

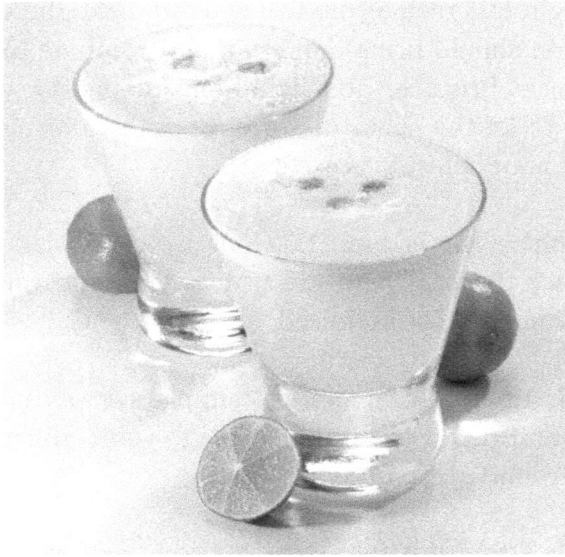

This is a fun cocktail that is going to give you a flavor that is so intense and so fresh that you will not be prepared for it thanks to the mixture of the lime and the mint. It is possible to make it an alcoholic drink with the pisco or to replace that with some sparkling water for those who just want something refreshing without the alcohol.

Ingredients

- 1 c. guava nectar
- 1 c. white rum or pisco (replace with sparkling water if going nonalcoholic).
- 2 tsp. superfine sugar
- Lime wedges
- Mint leaves
- Angostura bitters

Method

1. To start this simple recipe, take out a glass pitcher. Place the lime juice, sugar, guava nectar, and either the rum or the pisco.

2. Now you can add in a little bit of the Angostura bitters, as much as you would like and then stir the ingredients together well in order to let the sugar dissolve.

3. When ready to serve, divide up this mixture between 4 glasses of your choice. Add in the ice before topping with the mint and the lime wedge.

Place this drink into the fridge and let it cool down for a couple of hours before serving. This is better than using ice cubes because it allows the drink to be chilled without getting watered down from the ice.

Lemonade

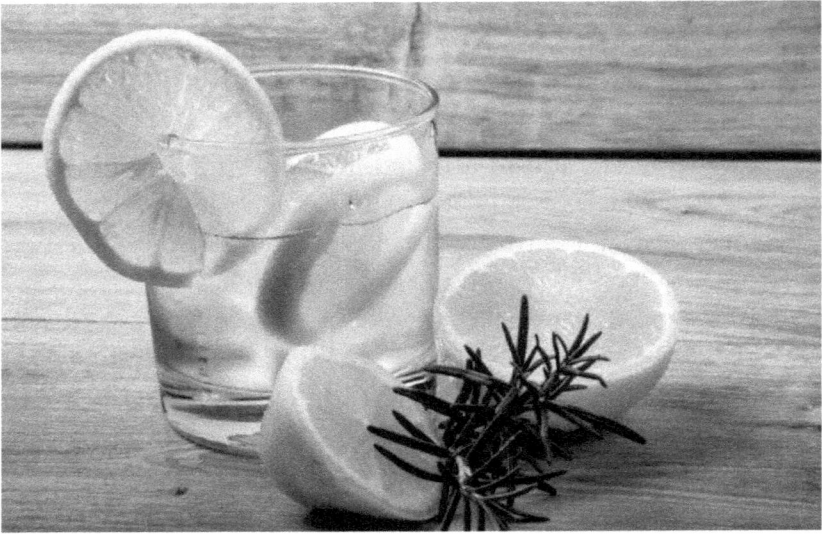

A classic favorite that everyone can remember from when they were kids. Whether you grew up in the Deep South or went to visit your grandmother in the country of the Midwest, there is always sure to be some great tasting lemonade available upon request. And now that you are all grown up, it is possible to try this new peach variety to get some of the old tastes that you enjoyed as a child with a new twist.

Ingredients

- ¾ c. sugar
- 1 c. lemon juice
- 3 c. cold water
- Lemon slices
- Ice cubes

Method

1. To begin this recipe, you can bring out a pitcher and add the sugar, lemon juice, and water. Stir this until the sugar has been completely dissolved

2. If you would like, place into the fridge to chill a bit. Serve over some ice and garnish with a few slices of lemon.

The recipe listed above is for the traditional lemonade that you grew up loving. A new way to produce this tasty drink is to add in some peachy flavor. To do this place half of a can of peach slices into the blender with a cup of your lemonade. Blend to get it smooth before pouring into the pitcher. Repeat with the rest of the peaches and then serve with some ice cubes.

Minty Iced Tea

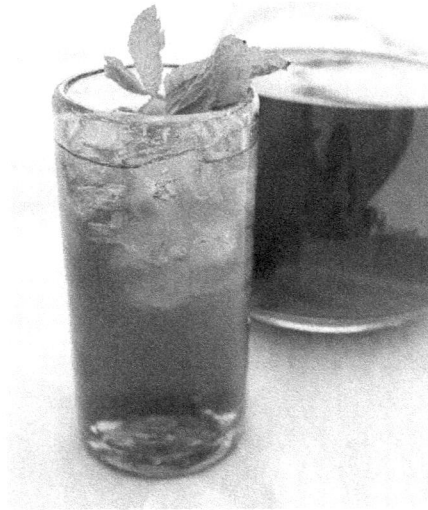

Tea just breathes the taste of summer and you will be able to get so many health benefits and great tastes when you use tea as the base ingredients. The next time that you are entertaining for the summer and need something cool and refreshing that everyone will enjoy, pull out this great recipe and be the hit of the party.

Ingredients

- 2 c. sugar
- 7 c. water
- 8 orange pekoe tea bags
- 8 c. water, cold
- 8 mint sprigs
- 2 c. orange juice
- Ice cubes
- Mint sprigs for garnish
- ¾ lemon juice

Method

1. First, take out a pan and combine the 7 cups of water with the 2 cups of sugar. Bring this to a boil and stir in the sugar to dissolve and then reduce the heat. Let this simmer for 5 minutes.

2. After this time, you can take it from the heat and add in the 8 sprigs of mint and the tea bags. Cover the pan and allow it stand for about 5 minutes. After this time remove the sprigs of mint and the tea bags with a spoon and discard them.

3. Transfer the heat to a big container before adding in the lemon juice, orange juice, and the remaining cold water.

4. Cover the bowl and let it set in the fridge for a minimum of 4 hours.

5. When you are ready to serve, place some ice in a few cups, pour the tea, and then garnish with mint sprigs if you would like.

This is a very large recipe of tea. If you are just serving for a smaller group and do not need as much tea, it is easy to halve the recipe to get the amount that you need.

Rose Collins

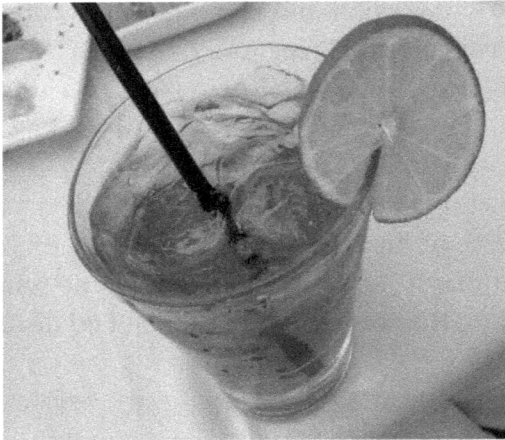

The first thing that you will notice about this drink is the floral smells and flavors that come with it. If it is a bit too girly for you, add a bit of Campari tames bitters in order to tame it all down to your preference.

Ingredients

- 3 Tbsp. vodka
- 2 Tbsp. rose syrup
- Lemon wheel, thin
- 1 tsp. Campari
- Chilled club soda and seltzer water
- Coarse sugar

Method

1. To start this recipe, bring out a cocktail shaker and combine the ice, Campari, rose syrup, and vodka. Shake for 30 seconds so that it is chilled.

2. When this is done, double strain it before placing into a Collins glass that is filled with ice. Top with the seltzer.

3. Right before you serve, float the lemon wheel into it and then sprinkle on the coarse sugar over it all.

If you are looking for a drink that is a little more sour and tart for your enjoyment, you can add in a bit of homemade sour mix. To make this sour mix, you can combine a simple syrup with lime juice and lemon juice in equal parts. Combine this in the cocktail shaker with the rest of the ingredients and then serve with this extra kick.

Tropical Smoothie

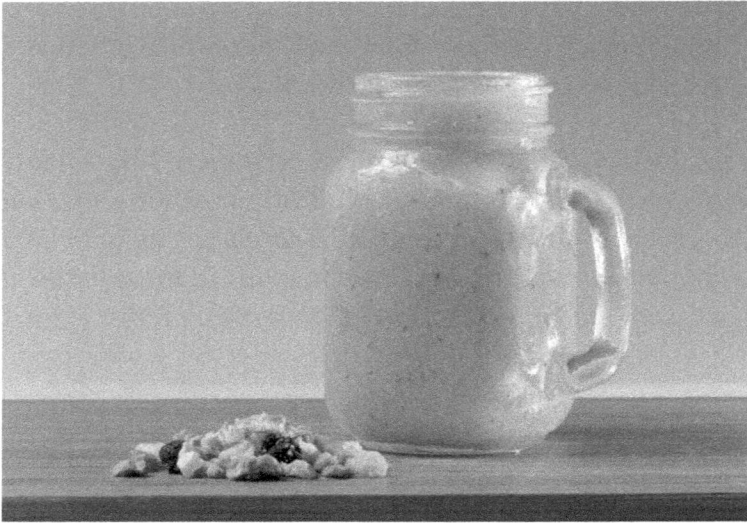

Take a vacation back to the islands this summer, even if you are stuck in the middle of the country. This is a great drink to enjoy either in the summer or in the winter and can give you a nice vacation away from it all.

Ingredients

- ½ c. chilled pineapple juice
- ½ frozen peeled bananas
- ½ c. chopped mango
- 1 Tbsp. lime juice
- ½ c. ice cubes

Method

1. For this recipe, you will need to bring out the blender. Place the lime juice, pineapple juice, banana, and mango inside.

2. Cover the blender and let it all blend so it becomes smooth. Slowly add in the ice and then continue to blend so you get the right consistency before serving.

You get to choose how creamy or smooth you would like the drink to be. If you like to have it with more of a juice like consistency, add in a few more ice cubes and blend for a bit longer. On the other hand, if you are interested in getting a smoother and creamier drink, add in a little bit more of the banana.

Coconut and Strawberry Cream Soda

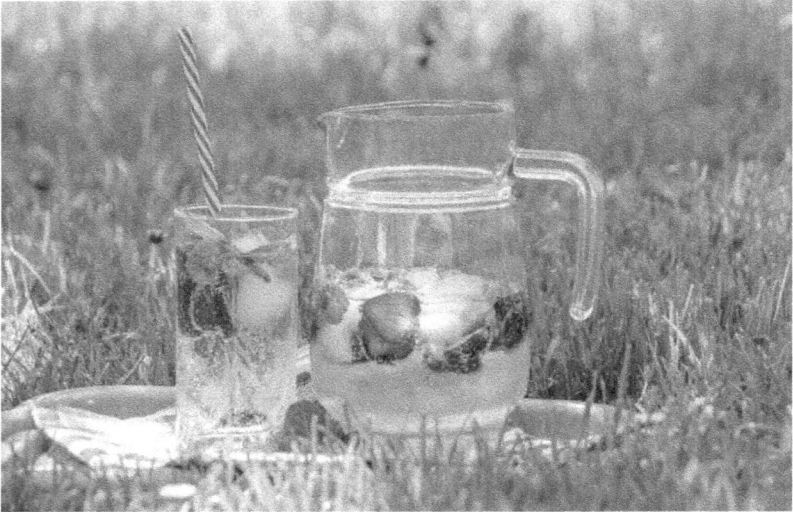

Coconut drinks are great because they can cool you down and get you all refreshed and ready to face the summer heat. You should look for some of the coconut milks in the grocery store to use for some of these delicious drinks.

Ingredients

- 2/3 c. sugar
- 3 c. halved strawberries
- 3 c. chilled carbonated water or club soda
- ¾ c. coconut milk, refrigerated.

Method

1. To begin this recipe, bring out a bowl and combine the sugar and the strawberries. Stir them well in order to cover the strawberries.

2. Once you are done with this, bring out a pastry blender and mash the strawberries coarsely.

3. Place about 1/3 cup of the berries into the bottom of six glasses. Add in some ice, a bit of club soda, and some coconut milk into each of the glasses.

4. Right before you are ready to serve, you can stir the drinks and then enjoy.

This is a great drink to have at a summer gathering or to cool off after working hard around the house or the garden. Double this recipe so that you have some stored up when needed. It is best to only store for a few days or you can freeze to get it to last a bit longer.

Carrot Lemonade

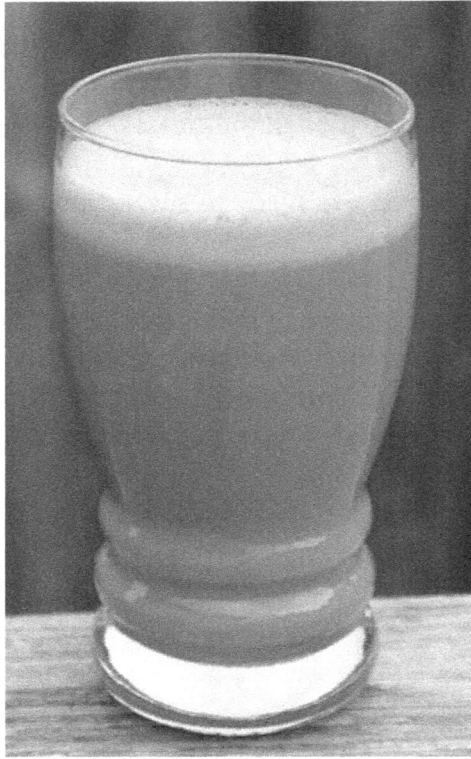

While the name might sound like it is a little bit out there, this lemonade is the one that you will need to make plenty of because the whole family will be asking for more. The best part is all of the healthy vitamins and minerals found inside that can keep your family strong and healthy for a long time to come.

Ingredients

- 2 c. water
- 1 lb. peeled and cut carrots
- ¾ c. lemon juice
- 3 c. pineapple juice

- Ice
- Cold water
- Lemon wedges

Method

1. Bring out a pan and combine the water and the carrots. Bring this to a boil before reducing the heat and covering it. Simmer these ingredients for about 30 minutes so the carrots can become tender.

2. When this is done, cool the mixture a bit before moving over to a blender. Add in a cup of the pineapple juice, cover the blender, and blend the ingredients until smooth.

3. Once the ingredients are the consistency that you would like, transfer to a plastic container allow to chill in the fridge for a few hours before serving.

This is a great way to sneak in some extra vegetables to your children's meals. This can be tricky but when the carrots are hidden, they will be begging for more. Look for sugar free pineapple juice in order to get some extra benefits out of the process.

Melon Heat Quenchers

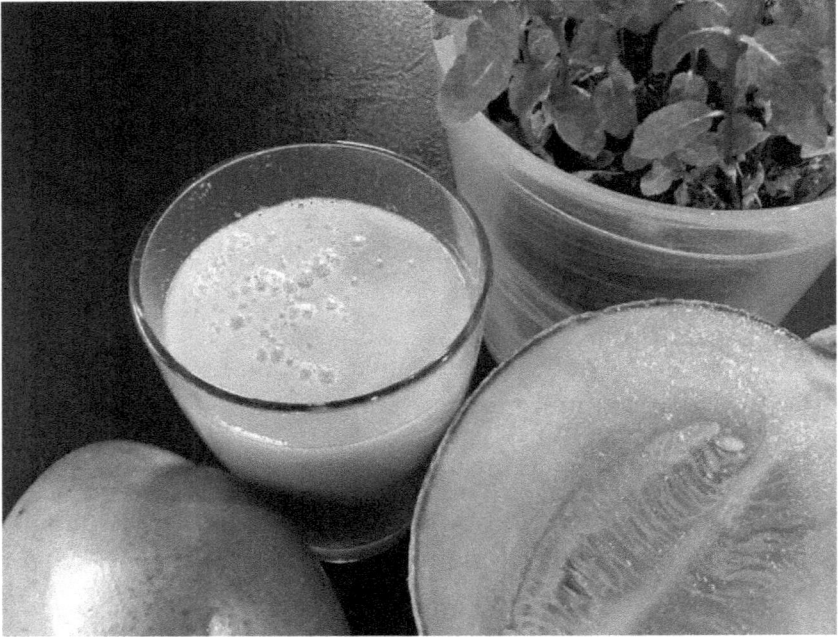

Melons come in so many different tastes and varieties that you are sure to find that one that will suit your mood. Check out this recipe and replace any melon that you want for something very unique.

Ingredients

- 3 ice cubes
- 1 c. watermelon, honeydew, or cantaloupe puree
- Plain yogurt
- ¼ grated ginger slice
- 1 tsp. honey
- Sparkling water (can have flavored if prefer)
- Lime peel, shredded

Method

1. To begin, puree the melon of your choice. To do this, chop up the melon and then place into a blender. Cover the blender and then turn on the machine to blend until fruit becomes smooth. You may need to stop a few times to push the mixture down and get it completely smooth.

2. Once that is done, add in the honey, a few teaspoons of yogurt, ginger, and ice cubes. Blend just to get the mixture smooth and frothy.

3. Pour this into a serving glass and add some more honey if you would like. Stir the lime peel next to taste and then fill up the rest of the glass with the sparkling water.

If you would like to add a little treat or snack to the drink you can make some melon skewers. To do this, you can scoop out the melon of your choice into little balls. Thread them onto the wooden skewers before laying on a baking sheet and freezing for a few hours. Serve with the drink.

Watermelon Punch

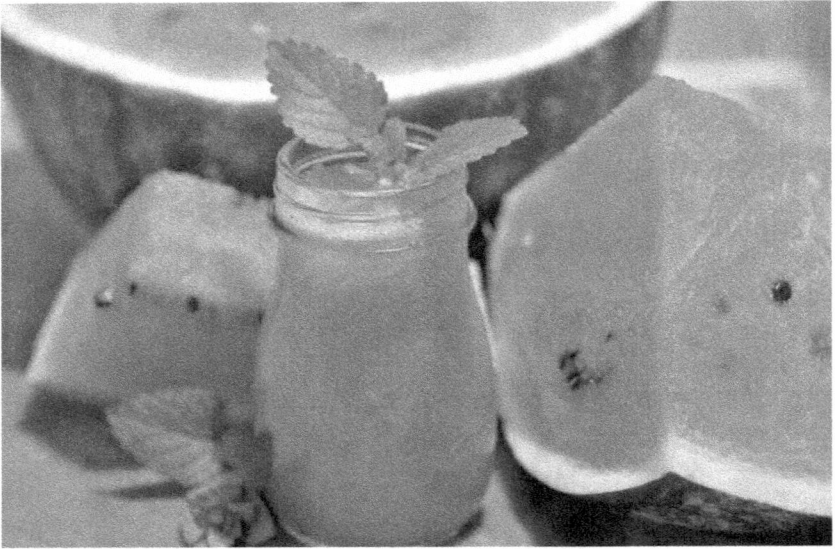

A tasty punch can spell the success of any summer day. Mixing a bit of watermelon with club soda, mint, sugar, lime juice, and white grape juice will give you the most festive drink you can find this summer in no time.

Ingredients

- ¾ c. watermelon
- 3 c. chopped and seeded watermelon
- ½ c. mint leaves, fresh
- 1 tsp. lime peel, shredded
- 2 c. white grape juice
- 32 oz. chilled club soda
- ¾ c. chilled lime juice
- Watermelon balls
- Mint sprigs

Method

1. To star this recipe, place the watermelon into a blender. Cover and let it blend for a few minutes so it becomes smooth. Strain this puree through a sieve and get rid of the pulp.

2. Take out a bowl and combine together the mint and the sugar. Use a wooden spoon to crush the mint and press it to the side of your bowl.

3. At this time, add in the watermelon puree, lime juice, lime peel, and grape juice. Stir these ingredients until the sugar has dissolved. Add in the club soda.

4. Pour this into glasses with some ice and garnish with the watermelon balls and mint sprigs before enjoying.

For a fun fruity taste, add in some more fruits to the juice. Strawberries and grapes are a great option but you can also use other types of melon for more flavor.

Raspberry Lemonade

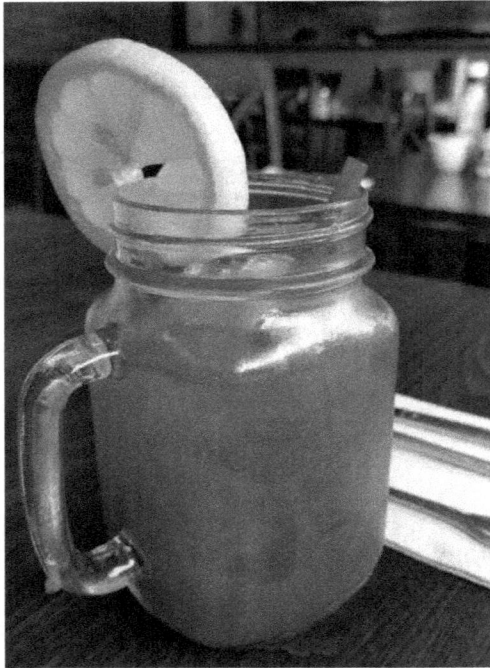

Nothing is as refreshing as a nice glass of lemonade when the summer heat gets to you, especially when you add in the light and fruity taste of raspberries. Keep a pitcher of this juice handy to enjoy whenever you get a hankering for the taste of summer.

Ingredients

- 12 oz. lemonade concentrate
- 18 oz. club soda
- 12 oz. vodka, pinnacle raspberry
- 1/8 c. grenadine
- Raspberries for garnish
- Lemon wedge, for garnish

Method

1. For this recipe, take out a pitcher and combine the regular ingredients together well.

2. Put the pitcher into the fridge and let it chill for a few hours before serving.

3. When you are ready to serve this juice, pour it into a few glasses that have ice in them and then enjoy.

When you do not have a measuring glass available, use the can for the lemonade concentrate to help with measuring. You will need one full can for the vodka amount and one and a half cans for the club soda amount.

Don't forget to share your thoughts on this book by leaving a review on Amazon.com. It takes just a few seconds.

Introduction to Green Smoothies (with 29 BONUS Green Smoothie Recipes)

We all know we should be getting more healthy greens in our diet and be eating more servings of fresh fruits and veggies. But the simple fact is most of us are just too busy to keep track of our diets as much as we would like to.

That's where green smoothies come in! With each recipe in this book, you'll get multiple servings of fruits AND veggies all in one easy to drink (and delicious) smoothie.

The average person needs a minimum of 2 cups of fruit and 2 ½ cups of vegetables each day. Most of these smoothie recipes will help you meet that requirement in just one smoothie!

The beauty of smoothies lies in their simplicity and their ability to disguise those veggies you might otherwise never eat. They're the perfect breakfast or midday snack. You can whip one up in less than 10 minutes and be on your way with a complete meal in a cup.

Unlike juices, smoothies allow you to get the fiber and other macronutrients from your fruits and veggies that are otherwise lost in the juicing process.

So, try out these recipes and don't be afraid to experiment and try out different variations of each recipe! With smoothies, the possibilities are endless!

The Spinach Surprise

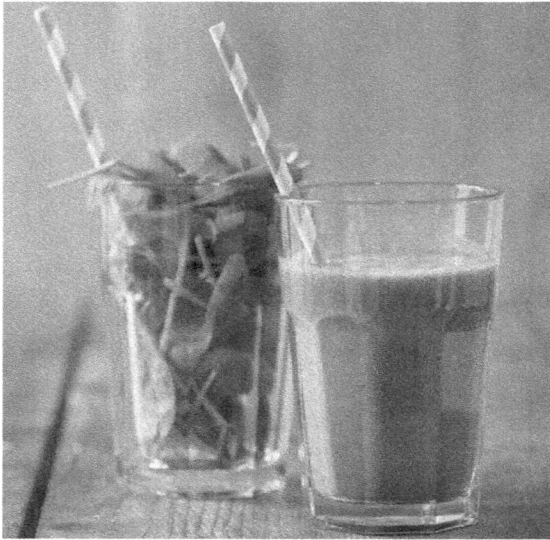

Ingredients

- 1 cup Spinach
- 1 cup Strawberries (chopped)
- 1 cup Plain Greek Yogurt
- 1 ripe Banana
- 1 Blood Orange (peeled, separated)
- 2 tsp Vanilla Extract
- 1 tsp Almond Oil

Method

1. Pulse together all ingredients until smooth. For a less thick smoothie, add whole milk and blend until it's your preferred thickness. For added protein and flavor, add a couple tablespoons of almond meal.

The Benefits

- The mild flavor of the spinach is perfectly masked by the powerfully sweet flavors of strawberries, banana, vanilla, and almond oil.

- No added sugar means you can consume this sweet treat totally guilt free!

- It also means you will save yourself from mood swings and energy crashes. This recipe provides quick but sustainable energy.

Power Boost

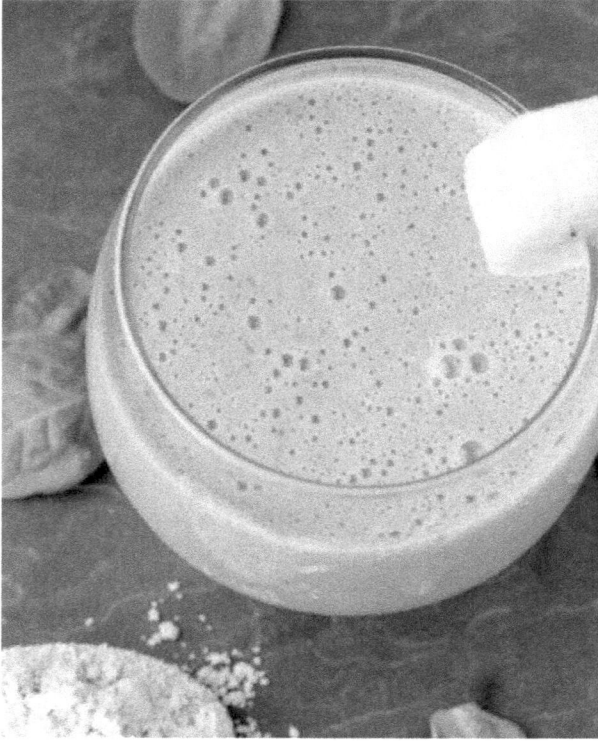

Ingredients

- 1 cup Spinach
- ½ cup Peanut Butter (or other nut butter)
- 1 cup Plain Greek Yogurt
- ½ cup Rolled Oats
- 2 ripe Bananas
- 1 Tbsp. Honey
- 1 tsp Vanilla Extract
- 2 tsp. Almond Oil

Method

1. Combine all ingredients in a blender and pulse until smooth. Serve in a bowl and top with chopped almonds and granola for added texture and protein.

The Benefits

- This smoothie contains 50 grams of protein, making it the perfect way to fill up and prevent between meal cravings.

- It also boasts 24 grams of fiber which will help boost your digestion and keep you energized.

- Eat this before a workout to improve your endurance and prevent muscle injury.

The Craving Killer

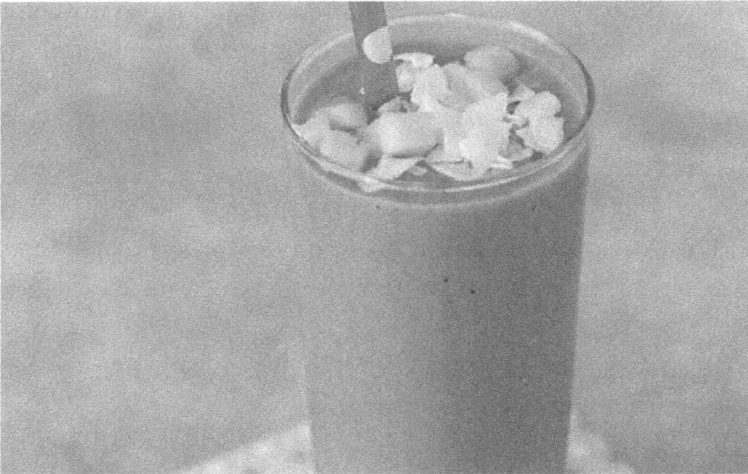

Ingredients

- 2 cups Spinach
- 1 cup Coconut Milk
- ½ cup Plain Greek Yogurt
- ½ cup Rolled Oats
- 1 Peach (chopped)
- 1 Mango (peeled, chopped)
- 3 Tbsps. Coconut Oil

Method

1. Blend ingredients together until smooth. Top with chopped almonds and coconut flakes for a little crunch.

2. If you aren't a huge fan of coconut, replace the coconut milk with whole milk (or another kind of full fat milk) and replace coconut oil with almond oil or olive oil.

The Benefits

- This smoothie is packed with healthy fats and natural fruit sugars which makes it the ultimate way to ward off pesky cravings for junk food.

- In addition to fighting cravings, the healthy fats combine with the vitamin E in the spinach to deeply nourish your skin and give you that youthful glow.

- The rich, bold tropical flavors of coconut, mango, and peach make it possible to double up on the spinach without risking that bitter after taste.

Green Morning

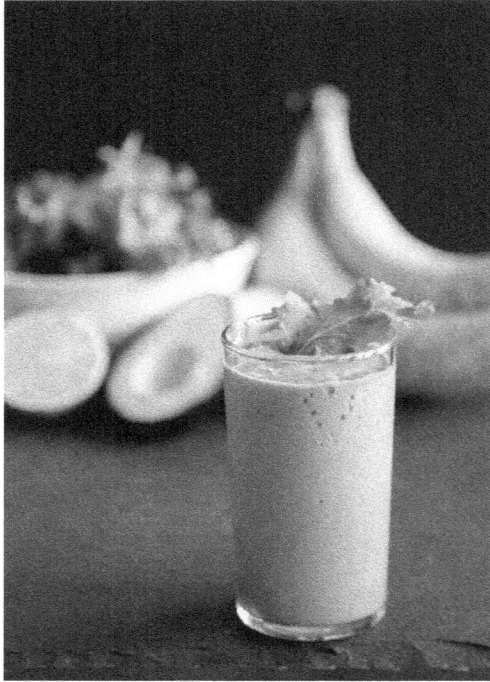

Ingredients

- ½ cup Spinach
- ½ cup Chard
- ¼ cup Fresh Basil
- 1 Avocado
- 1 ripe Banana
- 2 Apples
- 3 Kiwis
- ½ cup Plain Greek Yogurt
- 1 Tbsp. Honey (optional)
- 2 tsp Vanilla Extract

Method

1. Blend together the ingredients until smooth. Add whole milk as desired for a less thick smoothie.

2. The flavor of the greens are more pronounced in this recipe. If you're not yet ready to appreciate their flavors, add an orange and more vanilla extract to help mask the flavors.

The Benefits

- This recipe is a nutrient powerhouse that's especially rich in vitamin C, vitamin E, vitamin K, calcium, and potassium.

- This is the perfect substitute for that 2 o' clock cup of coffee or candy bar.

- It's got a great balance of fast-acting carbohydrate energy and slow-burning, long-lasting energy from protein and fiber.

The Ultimate All-in-One Smoothie

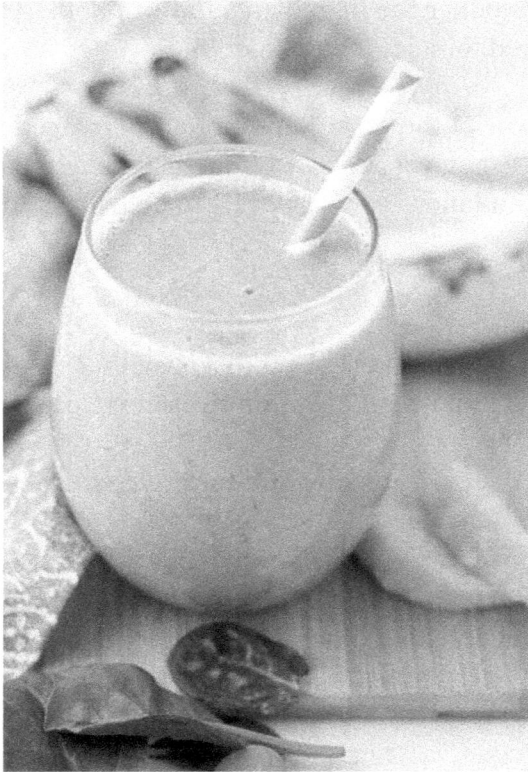

Ingredients

- 1 ½ cups Spinach
- 1 cup Carrots (chopped)
- 2 Peaches (chopped)
- 2 Oranges (peeled, separated)
- 2 Bananas
- ½ cup Rolled Oats
- ½ cup Plain Greek Yogurt
- ¼ cup Almond Meal

Method

1. Blend ingredients together until smooth. This will take a little longer with the carrot. Add whole milk as desired to make it less thick.

The Benefits

*   This smoothie contains all 9 servings of fruits and veggies that you need in a day!

*   The oats, yogurt, and almond meal provide some added protein, fiber, and healthy fats.

*   Make sure to drink this smoothie regularly throughout the summer. It's rich in beta carotenes and vitamin E which help protect the skin from sun damage.

Banana-Kale Burst

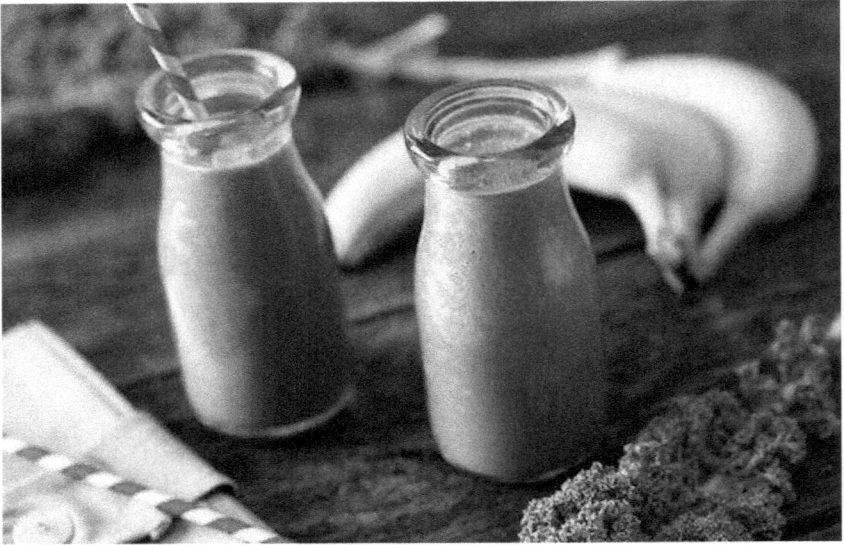

Ingredients

- 1 cup Kale (frozen)
- 1 ripe Banana
- 1 cup Plain Greek Yogurt
- 1 Apple (chopped)
- ¼ cup Coconut Milk
- 1 tsp Vanilla Extract
- 1 tsp Cinnamon

Method

1. Blend together all the ingredients until smooth. This can take a while with the kale (which may stay a little grainy even after blending well). If the kale taste is still too strong, add another banana.

The Benefits

- The kale in this recipe gives you all of your vitamin A, C, and K for the day.

- It's also rich in minerals like calcium, iron, and potassium.

- The banana adds even more potassium and quick energy in addition to the sweetness.

Protein Powerhouse

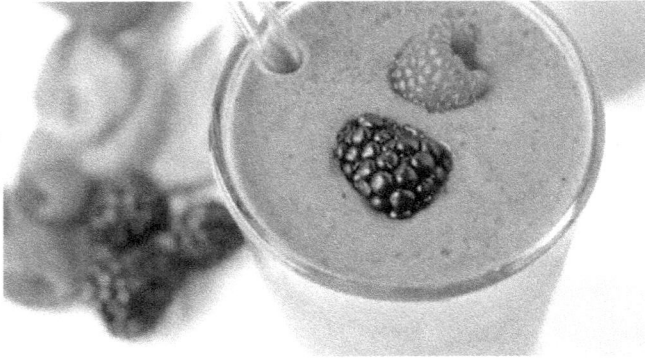

Ingredients

- 1 cup Kale
- 1 cup Spinach
- 1 cup Mixed Berries (frozen)
- 1 ripe Banana (frozen)
- 1 cup Rolled Oats
- ½ cup Almond Meal
- ¼ cup Almond Butter
- ½ cup Coconut Milk

Method

1. Blend the ingredients together until smooth. The blend of spinach and kale will help mellow out the bitterness of the kale. The frozen berries and banana add a cool, sweet slush.

The Benefits

- This smoothie packs more than 40 grams of protein so you'll be supercharged and ready to take on anything.

- All that protein is coming from highly nutritious sources so you're also getting a huge boost of vitamins and minerals.

- The high fiber content will help boost the metabolism and detox your body.

Inside and Out Smoothie

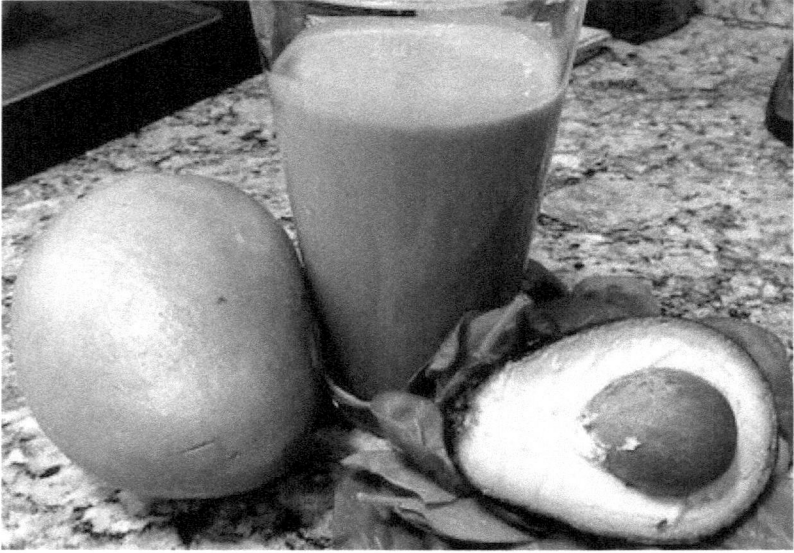

Ingredients

- 1 Avocado
- 1 cup Kale
- 2 Mangoes (peeled, chopped)
- ½ cup Coconut Milk
- ½ cup Plain Greek Yogurt
- 3-4 Tbsps. Almond Oil

Method

1. Blend everything together until smooth. The avocado, yogurt, milk, and oil will all help to create a smooth and creamy drink but you'll like still get some graininess from the kale.

The Benefits

- The nutrients in this smoothie will nourish and moisturize your skin in a way no lotion or facial mask ever could!

- The almond oil in this recipe will provide all your skin-nourishing vitamin E for the day.

- This recipe is also rich in healthy fats which help the skin keep its elasticity, preventing both wrinkles and cellulite.

The Friendly Green Giant

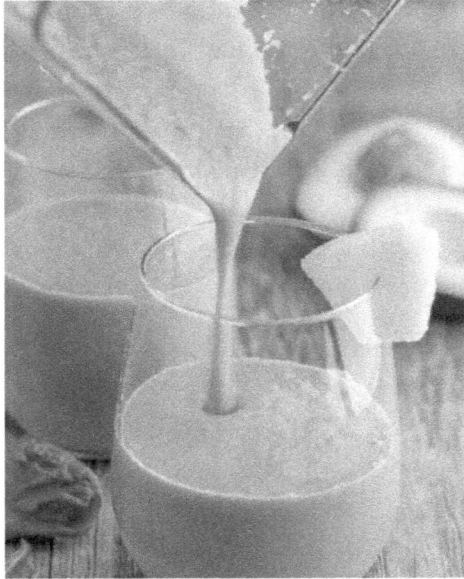

Ingredients

- 1 cup Kale
- 1 Avocado
- 1 cup Pineapple (chopped)
- 1"-2" Fresh Ginger (grated)
- 1 cup Plain Greek Yogurt
- ¼ cup Almond Meal
- 1 Tbsp. Honey (optional)

Method

1. Combine all the ingredients until smooth. The avocado will help add creaminess but you may still get some grain texture from the kale.

The Benefits

- The ginger is extremely effective for soothing many digestive problems from morning sickness and gas to diarrhea and loss of appetite so this is the perfect smoothie when you're not feeling well.

- Avocados are full of fiber and healthy fats which not only make them great for fighting cravings but also extremely beneficial to the heart.

- Pineapple has been shown to help keep teeth and gums healthy.

The Busy Morning Breakfast

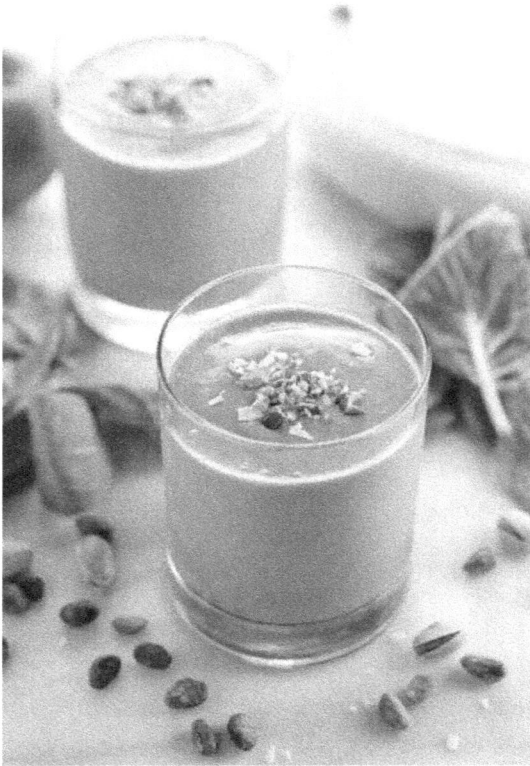

Ingredients

- 1 cup Kale
- 1 cup Spinach
- 1 Cucumber (frozen, chopped)
- 2 Peaches (chopped)
- 2 ripe Bananas (frozen)
- ½ cup Almond Butter
- ½ cup Whole Milk
- 1 tsp Vanilla Extract

Method

1. Blend ingredients together thoroughly. If the kale is too bitter for you, replace ½ cup of the kale with a ½ cup spinach. Use mangoes instead of peaches and coconut milk instead of regular for a more tropical feel.

The Benefits

- Get your 9 servings of fruits and veggies every day with this quick and delicious recipe.

- In addition to getting all your fruits and veggies, you're also getting a great amount of protein, fiber, and healthy fats making this a perfect meal replacement.

- The nutrients in this recipe can help strengthen the immune system, improve heart health, and stabilize your blood sugar levels.

An Avocado Dream

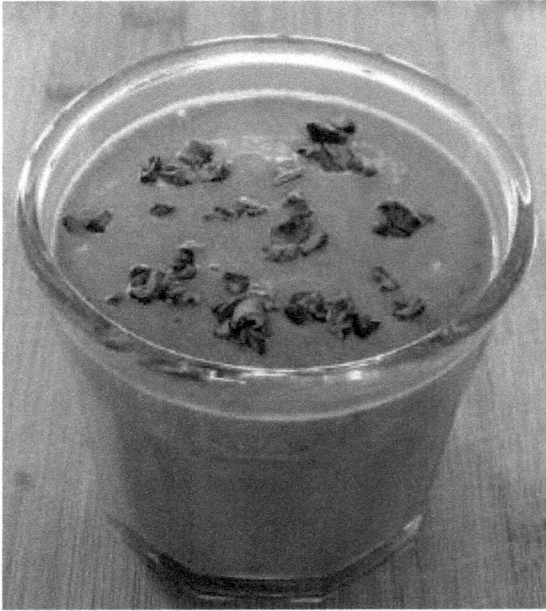

Ingredients

- 2 Avocadoes
- 1 cup Coconut Milk
- ½ cup Dark Cherries (pitted)
- ½ cup Almond Meal
- 1 Tbsp. Almond Oil
- ¼ cup Dark Chocolate Chips
- Crushed Ice

Method

1. In a double boiler, melt chocolate over medium heat. Once melted, combine it with the rest of the ingredients in the

blender until smooth. Add crushed ice until you get your desired consistency.

2. This rich, silky smoothie feels and tastes great. Serve it in a bowl topped with crushed almonds, dark chocolate chips, and dried cherries.

The Benefits

- Dark chocolate and dark cherries are both extremely rich in antioxidants.

- Avocadoes and almond oil are rich in healthy fats that are great for your heart and your skin.

- This recipe is also a great source of fiber and protein.

Endurance Booster

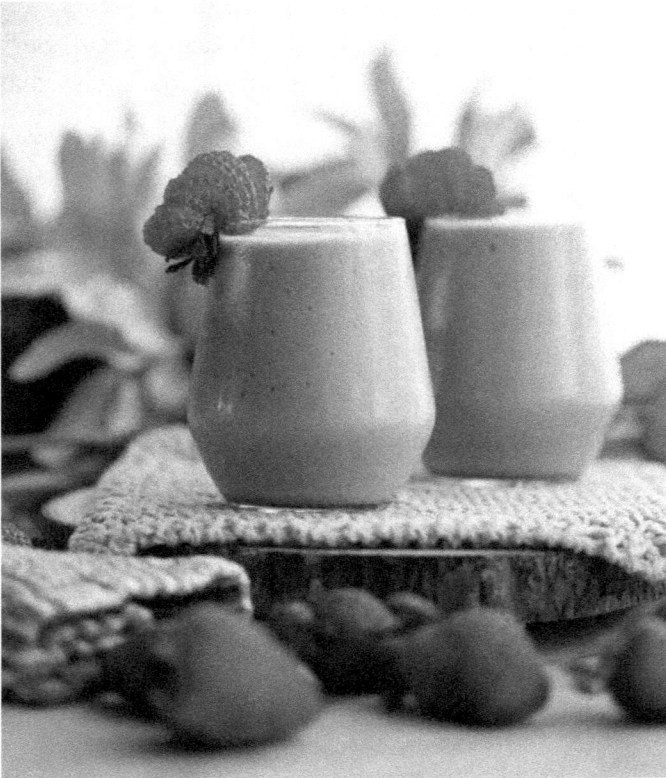

Ingredients

- 1 Avocado
- 1 cup Spinach
- 1 cup Strawberries (frozen, chopped)
- ½ cup Peanut Butter
- ½ cup Plain Greek Yogurt
- ¼ cup Almond Meal
- 1 tsp Vanilla Extract
- 1 tsp Cinnamon

Method

1. Blend ingredients together until smooth and silky.

The Benefits

- This recipe boasts more than 40 grams of protein, helping you to stay energized and build muscle.

- The protein in combination with the healthy fats in this recipe help add gloss to your hair and a youthful glow to your skin.

- The strawberries are an amazing source of antioxidants.

The Fat Burner

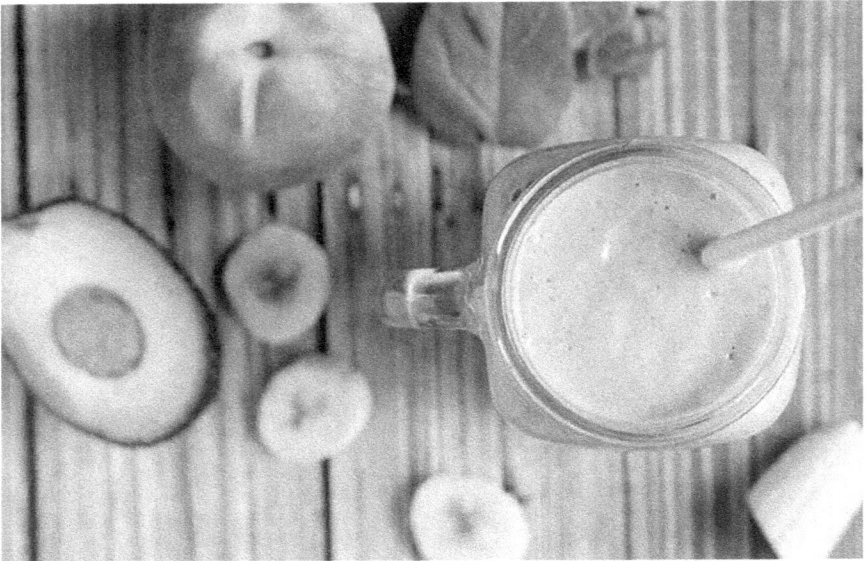

Ingredients

- 2 Avocadoes
- 2 ripe Bananas (frozen, chopped)
- 1 large Peach (chopped)
- 1 large Carrot (chopped)
- ½ cup Almond Butter
- 1 cup Coconut Milk
- 1 tsp Vanilla Extract

Method

1. Blend ingredients together until smooth. This may take longer with the carrot.

The Benefits

- The perfect balance of protein, fiber, and healthy fats makes this an amazing metabolism booster and craving killer at the same time!

- The high beta-carotene content helps protect your skin from sun damage and prevent damage to the eyes.

- The high potassium helps lower blood pressure.

Green Fuel

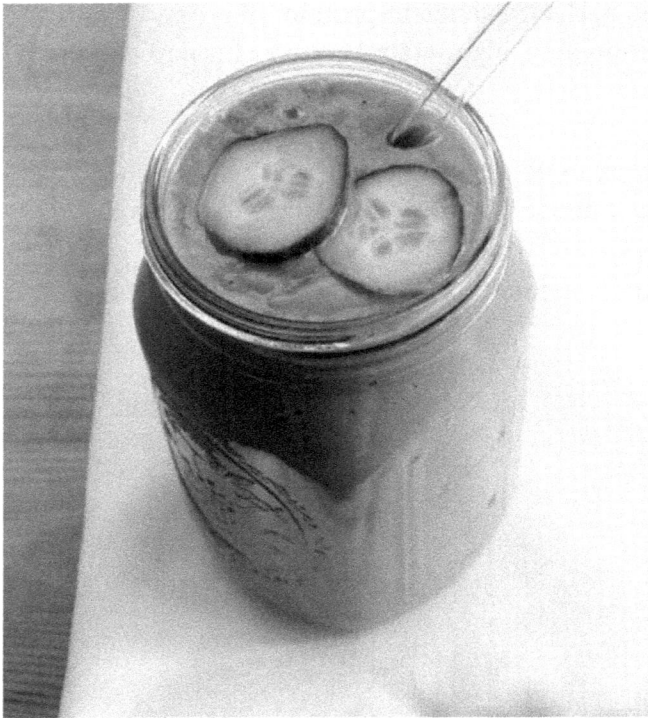

Ingredients

- 2 cups Spinach
- 1 Avocado
- 1 Cucumber (frozen)
- 1 Banana (frozen)
- 2 Kiwis
- 1 Apple
- ½ cup Plain Greek Yogurt
- ½ cup Whole Milk
- 2 tsp Vanilla Extract

Method

1. Blend ingredients together until smooth.

The Benefits

- This recipe is rich in vitamin C, E, and K.

- It's also packed with potassium, calcium, and iron.

- The high fiber content will detox your system, preventing acne breakouts and evening your skin tone.

All You Need Smoothie

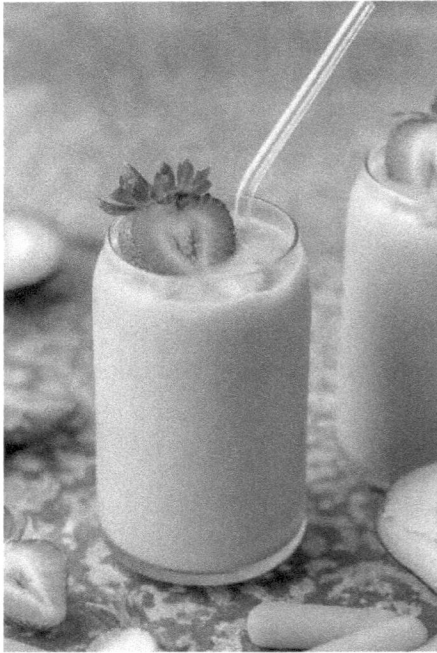

Ingredients

- 1 Avocado
- 1 cup Spinach
- ½ cup Chard
- ½ cup Kale
- ½ cup Carrots (chopped)
- 1 cup Strawberries
- 1 ripe Banana
- 1 Orange
- ½ cup Coconut Milk
- ½ cup Plain Greek Yogurt
- 2 tsp Vanilla Extract

Method

1. Combine all ingredients together in a blender until smooth.

The Benefits

- This smoothie takes the stress out of healthy eating by providing all 9 servings of fruits and veggies in one glass!

- You're also getting all your vitamin A, C, and K for the day.

- This smoothie is also filled to the brim with antioxidants.

Sweet Spirulina Magic

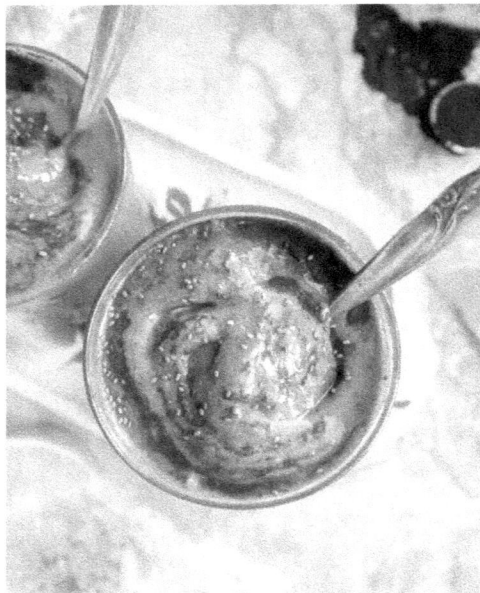

Ingredients

- 1 Mango
- 1 small Lemon (peeled, seeded)
- ½ cup Spinach
- 1 Tbsp. Spirulina Powder
- 1 ripe Banana
- ½ cup Coconut Milk
- ½ cup Plain Greek Yogurt

Method

1. Blend all ingredients together. The spirulina will turn this smoothie a dramatic green color but don't let that stop you from enjoying the taste.

The Benefits

- Spirulina is a superfood. It contains a full range of vitamins and minerals.

- Believe it or not, it's also an amazing source of protein!

- This recipe is a great way to introduce spirulina into your diet. As you get used to it, up the amount of spirulina you add.

The Ultimate Workout Fuel

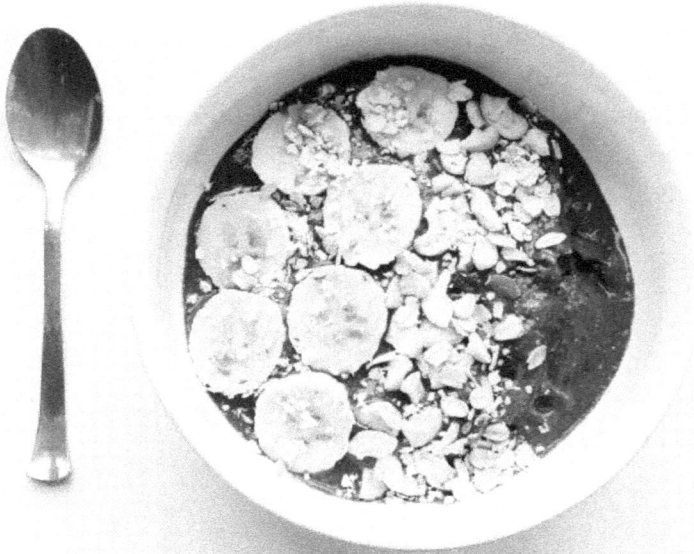

Ingredients

- ½ cup Oatmeal
- ½ cup Almond Meal
- ¼ cup Almond Butter
- 2 Tbsps. Spirulina Powder
- 2 Bananas
- ½ cup Plain Greek Yogurt
- ¼ cup Whole Milk
- ¼ cup Dark Chocolate Chips

Method

1. Blend ingredients together until smooth. For a richer chocolate flavor, melt the dark chocolate in a double boiler before adding it to the smoothie.

2. Serve in a bowl topped with chopped almonds and dark chocolate chips.

The Benefits

*   This is an extremely high protein smoothie that also packs a lot of other nutrients as well.

*   Improve endurance and decrease muscle soreness by drinking this before workouts.

*   The spirulina and chocolate are rich in key antioxidants.

The Body Sculptor

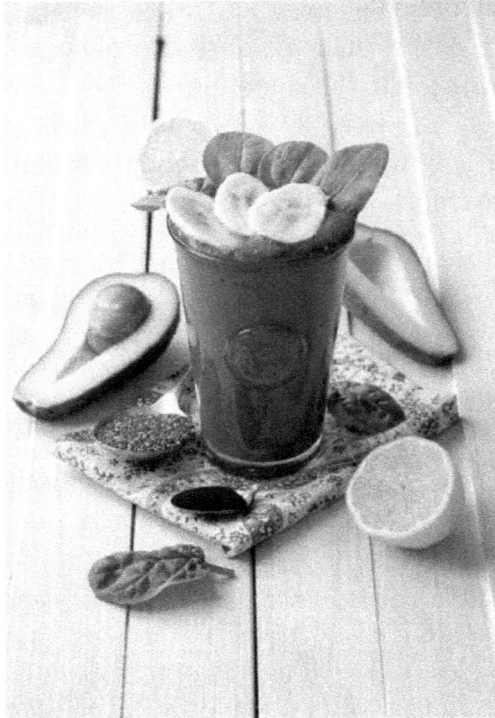

Ingredients

- 1 Avocado (frozen)
- 2 Tbsps. Spirulina Powder
- 2 Bananas (frozen)
- 1 Orange
- 1 Mango
- 2 Tbsps. Almond Oil
- ½ cup Coconut Milk
- ½ cup Whole Milk
- 1 tsp Vanilla Extract

Method

1. Blend ingredients together until smooth. Replace whole milk with plain Greek yogurt for a thicker smoothie.

The Benefits

- Avocado and almond oil provide healthy unsaturated fats that help kill cravings and burn fat.

- Spirulina and orange provide immune system boosting vitamin C.

- Vitamin C also helps detox and clear up blemished skin.

Looking Good in Green

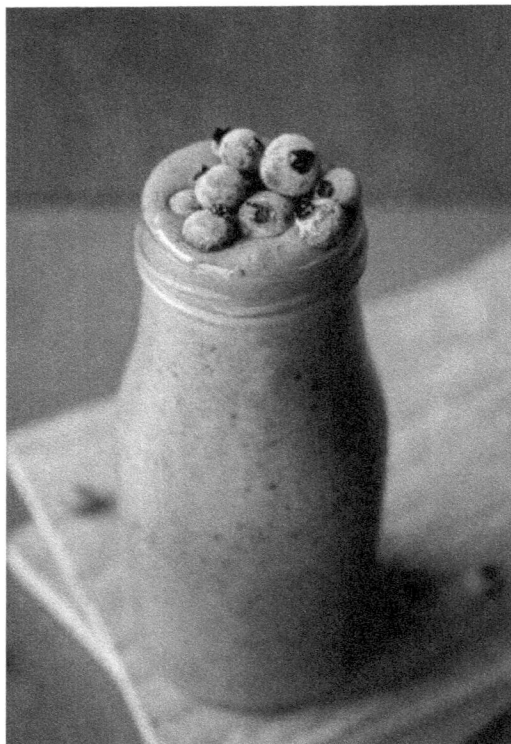

Ingredients

- 1 Avocado
- 1 cup Spinach
- 2 Tbsps. Spirulina Powder
- 2 Kiwis
- ½ cup Blueberries (frozen)
- ½ cup Blackberries (frozen)
- ½ cup Whole Milk
- ½ cup plain Greek Yogurt
- 2 tsp Vanilla Extract

Method

1. Combine ingredients in a blender until smooth. The softer the kiwi, the sweeter it will be so use extremely ripe kiwis to avoid needing added sugar.

The Benefits

- This smoothie is supercharged with antioxidants from the berries, kiwis, and spirulina.

- Kiwis contain more vitamin C than oranges.

- Spinach, yogurt, and milk help provide a high dose of calcium.

On the Go Smoothie

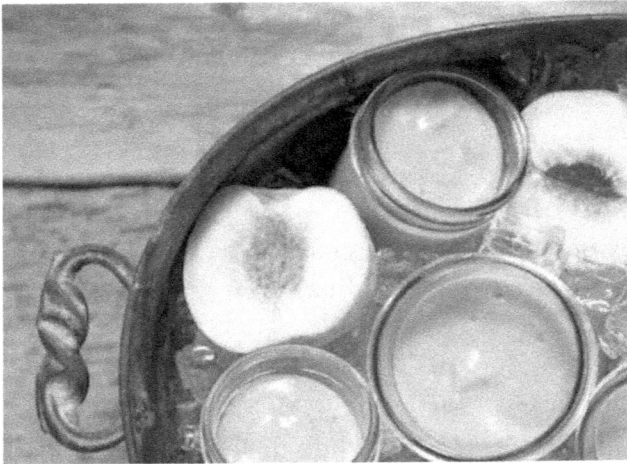

Ingredients

- 1 large Cucumber (frozen)
- 1 cup Spinach
- 2 Peaches
- 1 Apple
- 2 large Carrots
- 2 Tbsps. Spirulina Powder
- ½ cup plain Greek Yogurt
- ½ cup Whole Milk
- 2 tsp Vanilla Extract

Method

1. Blend ingredients together until smooth. Replace the yogurt with milk for a more easy-to-drink beverage. Replace the milk with yogurt for a thicker, more satisfying meal replacement.

The Benefits

- With all 9 servings of fruits & veggies, this smoothie is perfect for those who don't have the time to cook complete, balanced meals each day.

- This recipe is packed with all of your essential vitamins and minerals. Try drinking this instead of taking a multi-vitamin!

- The high fiber content in this smoothie will help lower blood pressure, speed up your metabolism and fight cravings.

Berry-Celery Swirl

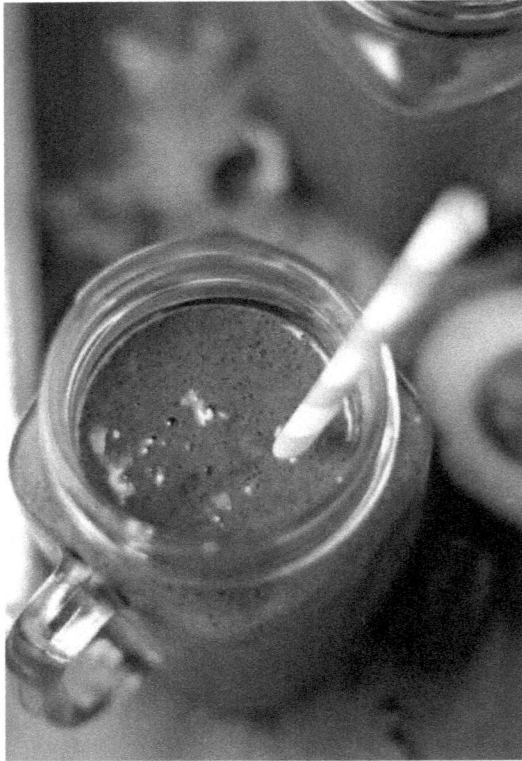

Ingredients

- ½ cup Strawberries
- ¼ cup Blueberries
- ¼ cup Raspberries
- 2 large Celery Stalks
- 1 Tbsp. Spirulina
- ½ cup Coconut Milk
- ½ cup plain Greek Yogurt
- 2 tsp Vanilla Extract

Method

1. Blend ingredients together until smooth. The celery may not grind completely smooth.

The Benefits

- Celery is a great source of fiber and many minerals.

- While it used to be considered a nutrient-poor vegetable, celery is now known to be packed with many key antioxidants.

- Celery contains a compound (apiuman) which strengthens your stomach lining and prevents ulcers.

Peanut Butter Celery Energy Booster

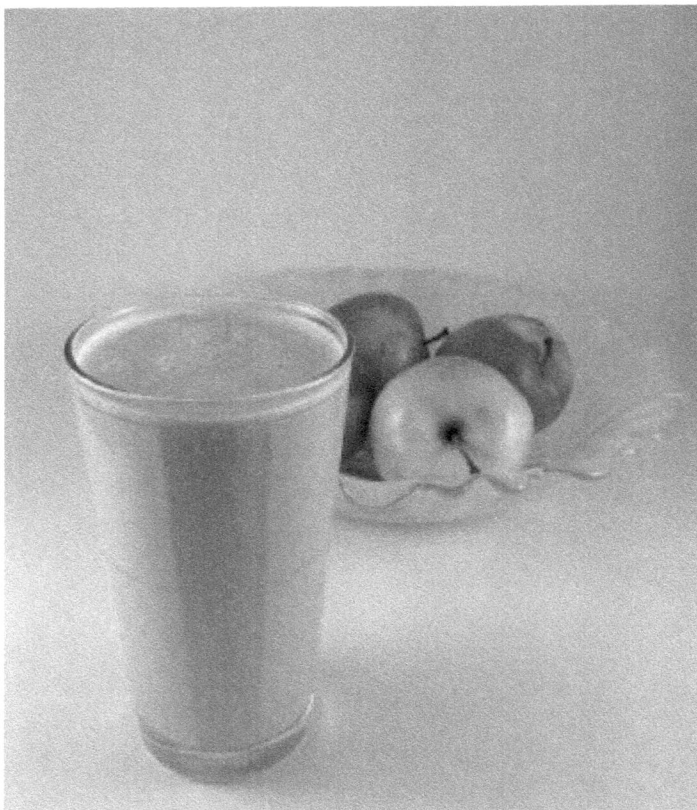

Ingredients

- 3 large Celery Stalks
- ½ cup Peanut Butter (or Almond)
- ½ cup Hazelnut Paste
- 2 Apples
- 1 Cucumber (frozen)
- 1 cup Whole Milk
- 1 Tbsp. Honey

Method

1. Blend ingredients together until smooth.

The Benefits

-   This recipe takes the classic celery and peanut butter combo and transforms it into the ultimate protein boost.

-   Hazelnuts have been shown to help lower bad cholesterol.

-   This smoothie is high in magnesium and calcium, both of which help to repair and strengthen muscles.

Soothing Celery Smoothie

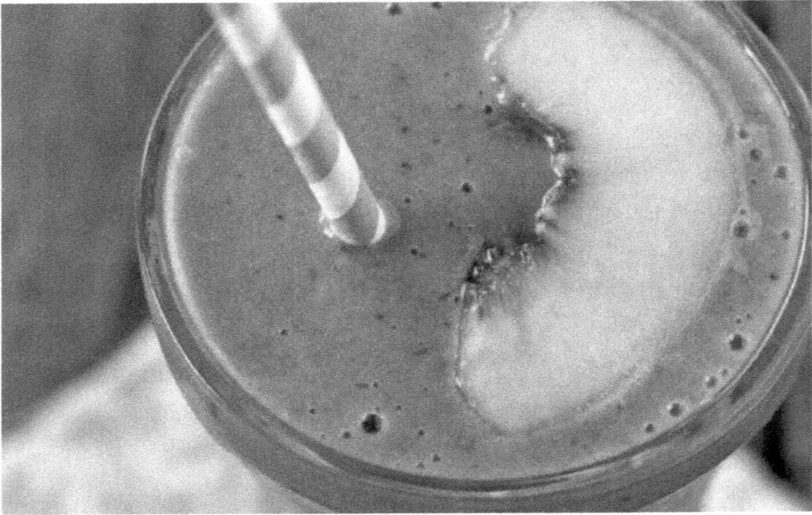

Ingredients

- 2 large Celery Stalks
- ½ cup Spinach
- 2 Peaches
- ½ cup Hazelnut Paste
- ½ cup Almond Butter
- ½ cup Coconut Milk
- ½ cup Whole Milk
- 2 Tbsps. Almond Oil
- 1 tsp Vanilla Extract

Method

1. Combine all ingredients together in a blender until smooth. This can take a while with celery.

The Benefits

- The oils found in the hazelnuts and almonds help lower cholesterol and slow the ageing process in your skin.

- This recipe is high in fiber which will help detox your body and burn fat.

- Most ingredients are loaded with minerals which help build strong bones and muscles.

The Green Detox

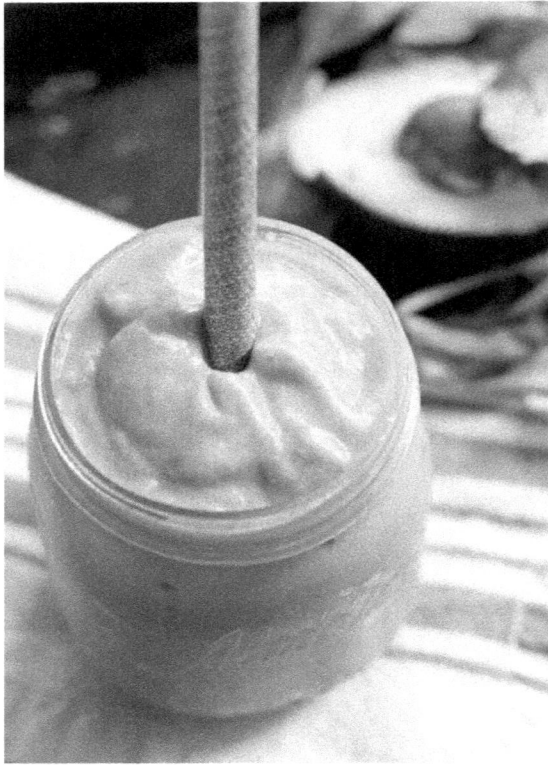

Ingredients

- 1 Avocado
- 2 large Celery Stalks
- ½ cup Spinach
- 2 Kiwis
- 1 Apple
- 1 Banana
- 1 cup Coconut Milk

Method

1. Blend ingredients together until smooth. Replace coconut milk with regular whole milk if you aren't a fan of coconut flavor.

The Benefits

- The high lauric acid content of coconut milk has been found to help treat both viral and bacterial infections.

- This recipe is rich in anti-inflammatory compounds which can help even skin tone and manage arthritic joint pain.

- Many ingredients are also rich in vitamin C and antioxidants.

Nourish the Body & Mind

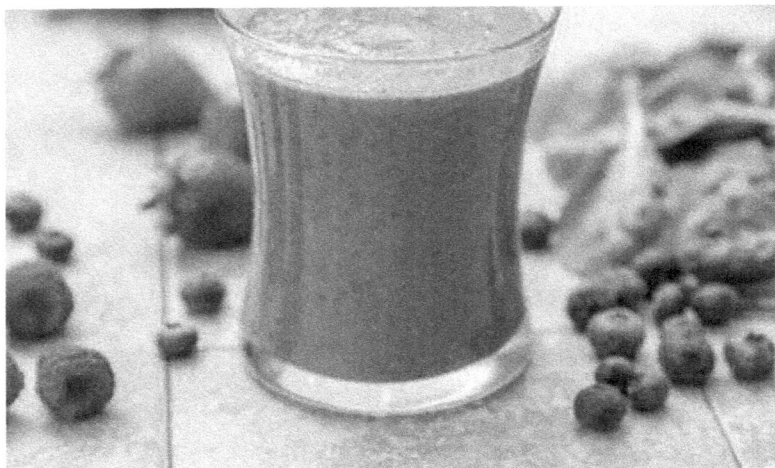

Ingredients

- 1 cup Spinach
- 2 large Celery Stalks
- ½ cup Kale
- 1 cup Blueberries
- ½ cup Strawberries
- ½ cup Blackberries
- ½ cup Coconut Milk
- ½ cup Plain Greek Yogurt
- 1 Tbsp. Almond Oil
- 1 tsp Vanilla Extract

Method

1. Blend all ingredients together until smooth. This could take a while with the kale and celery.

The Benefits

- This smoothie boasts a complete nutrition profile with all 9 servings of your fruits & veggies for the day.

- With 2 cups of berries, you're getting a huge dose of skin-protecting antioxidants.

- The greens in this recipe are full of iron, calcium, and magnesium.

Bold Pineapple Chard Breakfast

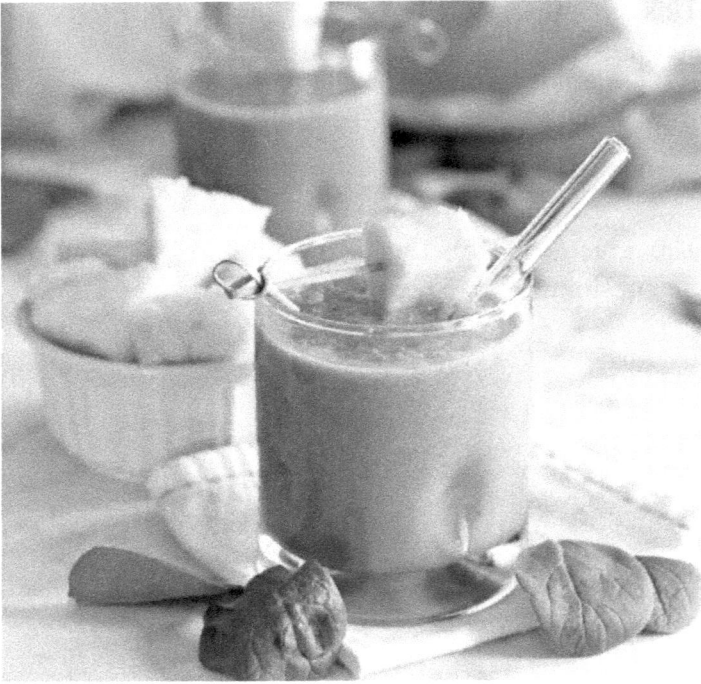

Ingredients

- 1 cup Chard
- ½ cup Spinach
- 1 cup Pineapple Chunks
- 1 cup Coconut Milk
- 1 Mango
- 1 Banana

Method

1. Blend all ingredients together until smooth.

The Benefits

- It may not have the prettiest name but chard contains high amounts of at least 13 different antioxidants!

- That includes syringic acid which slows down the rate at which your body breaks down carbs (meaning you get a steady stream of energy rather than a sudden burst).

- This slower break down of carbs also means you'll be able to use more of that energy rather than just store it as fat—as your body usually does with the excess carbs.

Afternoon Pick-Me-Up

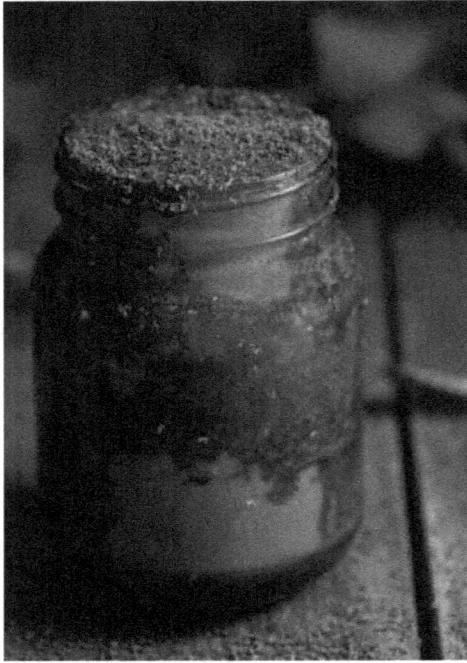

Ingredients

- 1 cup Chard
- 1 Tbsp. Spirulina Powder
- ½ cup Almond Butter
- ½ cup Rolled Oats
- ¼ cup Dark Chocolate Chips
- 1 cup Whole Milk
- 1 Banana

Method

1. Combine all ingredients together in a blender until smooth.

The Benefits

- Almond butter, oats, and spirulina combine to provide a major protein boost more powerful than any cup of coffee.

- Dark chocolate adds even more antioxidants to the 13 already found in the chard.

- Banana and milk help provide an immediate energy boost while you wait for the protein to kick in.

Chard Cleanser

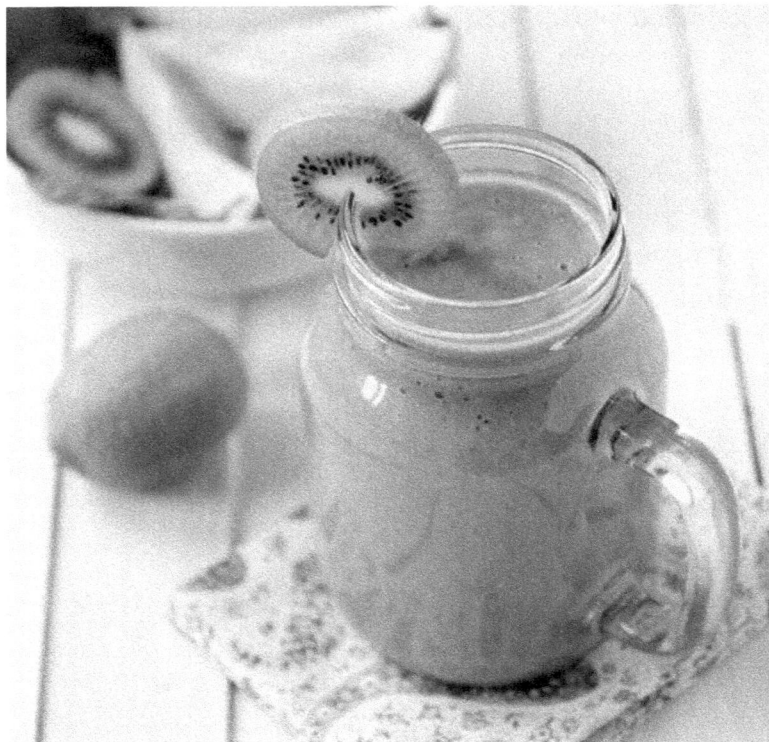

Ingredients

- 1 cup Chard
- 1 cup Rolled Oats
- ½ cup Spinach
- 1 large Carrot
- 1 Orange
- 1 Mango
- 2 Kiwis
- 2 Tbsps. Almond Oil
- 1 cup Coconut Milk

Method

1. Blend all ingredients together until smooth.

The Benefits

- This smoothie is packed with fiber and healthy fats which work together to detox the body and nourish you from head to toe.

- The fats, vitamins, and minerals in coconut milk and almond oil help hydrate your skin from the inside out.

- The antioxidants in the fruits and veggies help protect your cells from damage, keeping you looking and feeling young.

Going Green

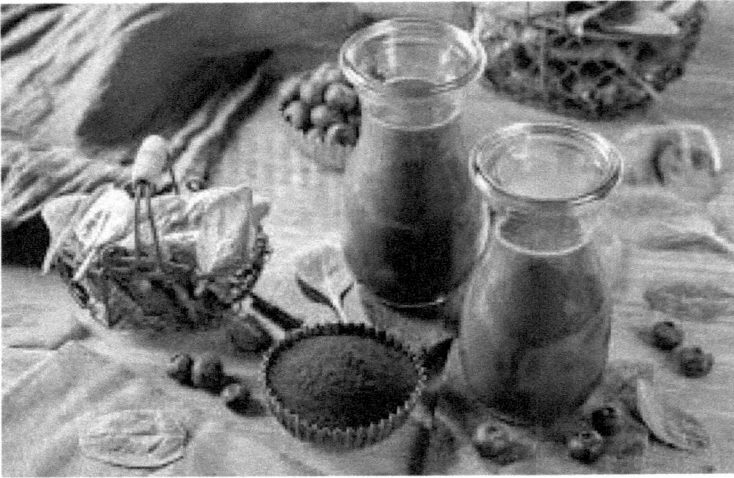

Ingredients

- 1 cup Chard
- 1 cup Spinach
- ½ cup Blueberries
- 1 Tbsp. Spirulina Powder
- 2 Kiwis
- 1 Apple
- 1 Lime (seeded)
- 2 ripe Bananas
- 1 cup Whole Milk

Method

Combine ingredients in a blender until smooth. Add plain Greek yogurt to thicken it or crushed ice for a chilled, slushy beverage.

The Benefits

- The combination of fruits and veggies in this recipe provide a full spectrum of vitamins and minerals.

- It also has a high fiber content making it perfect for those trying to lose some extra weight.

- The protein in the milk and spirulina powder provide a nice kick to get you motivated.

Discover Scientifically-Proven "Shortcuts" & "Hacks" to Lose Weight FASTER (With Very Little Effort)

For this month only, you can get Linda's best-selling & most popular book absolutely free – *Weight Loss Secrets You NEED to Know*.

Get Your FREE Copy Here:
TopFitnessAdvice.com/Bonus

Discover scientifically-proven tips to help you lose weight faster and easier than ever before. With this book, readers were able to improve their weight loss results and fitness levels. So, it's highly recommended that you get this book, especially while it's free!

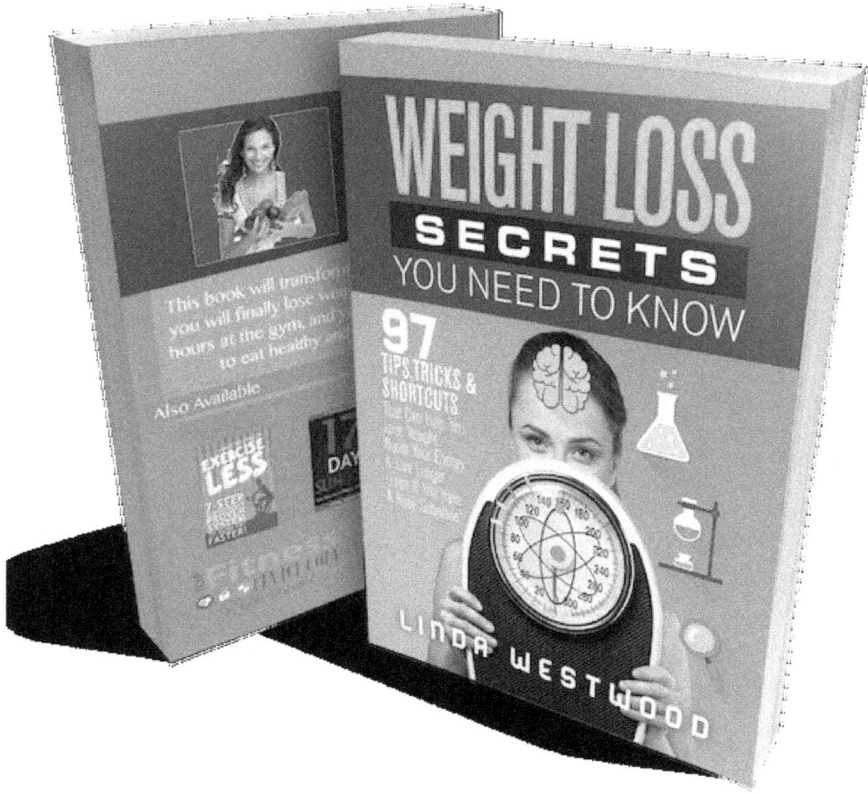

Get Your FREE Copy Here:

TopFitnessAdvice.com/Bonus

Final Words

I would like to thank you for purchasing my book and I hope I have been able to help you and educate you on something new.

If you have enjoyed this book and would like to share your positive thoughts, could you please take 30 seconds of your time to go back and give me a review on my Amazon book page.

I greatly appreciate seeing these reviews because it helps me share my hard work.

You can leave me a review on Amazon.com

Again, thank you and I wish you all the best!

Enjoying this book?

Check out my other best sellers!

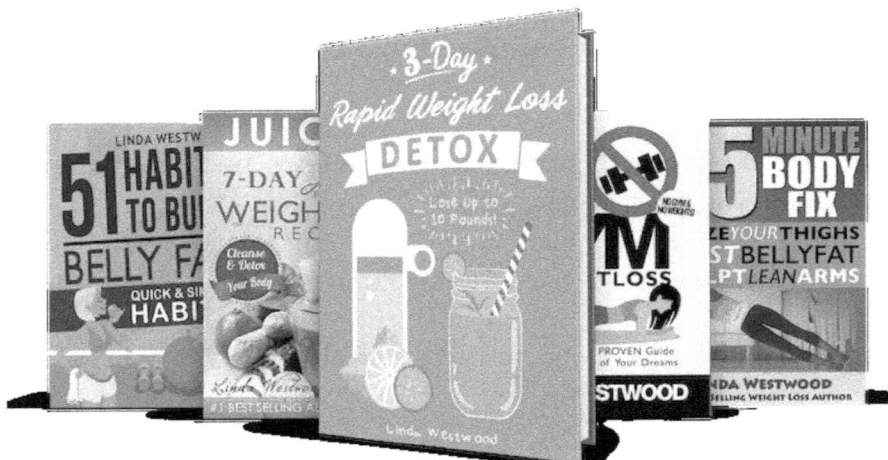

www.ingramcontent.com/pod-product-compliance
Lightning Source LLC
Chambersburg PA
CBHW031143020426

42333CB00013B/489